FIERCE

—— and ——

FABULOUS

—— after ——

MENOPAUSE

Unleash the Power of Midlife Change to
Rediscover Your Purpose, Reignite Your Passions,
and Reclaim Your Authentic Self

LYDIA TAYLOR

Contents

It's easy to get caught up in life.
To get ravelled up in the loud expectations of how you should act,
what you should want
and who you should be.

And before you know it, it's as if you're in the middle of a huge ball of
wool, surrounded by layer upon layer of noise.

Noise that is not yours. A voice that is not yours.

We often talk about self-discovery
But actually, I think it's self-uncovery.

You need to uncover the person who has always been there right at the
center, right at the core of that ball of wool.
Before you got so tied up in what everyone else thought you should be.

So it's ok to unravel sometimes. To start peeling back those layers of
noise that have surrounded you for so long.

And when you're done, listen carefully.
You will hear something you probably haven't heard for a long time. A
familiar noise but one that you cannot place.

That's the sound of you.

You. Without the expectations of every could-be, would-be, should-be
that's ever been handed to you.

You.

Sit with that sound for a while.
It might feel a lot like silence.

But sit a while longer and listen a little harder.
And you'll realize that, actually …

It feels a lot like peace.

-- Becky Hemlsey, Poet

Introduction: From Aunt Flo to the Menopause Show

Beloved stand-up comedian Joan Rivers once joked,

> *"A study says owning a dog makes you 10 years younger. My first thought was to rescue two more, but I don't want to go through menopause again."*

Welcome to the book on menopause we all wish we had sooner! I want to kick things off with a bit of a narrative twist. You see, when it comes to menopause, it's often portrayed as a gloomy story —one marked by the loss of our youth, fertility, and purpose. But what if we turned the tables on that narrative? What if, instead of dwelling on what's left behind, we viewed menopause as an exciting tale of growth—a phase where we wholeheartedly embrace wisdom, confidence, and a fresh sense of purpose like never before? Sounds like more fun to me!

Now, let's get down to brass tacks. Menopause is never a breeze— although we do appreciate those cool drafts more often as we welcome the soul-sucking hot flashes that could rival volcanic eruptions into our lives. Don't get me started on night sweats that could leave a bathmat dripping or those surprise acne breakouts that make us feel like we're back in high school, applying Clearasil every hour. Weight gain? Please, that menopause muffin top is no joke.

Did I mention we miss sex, or even having the desire? We're missing intimacy and human touch, but we dare not discuss it. The absence of closeness is messing with our relationships and leaving us questioning our ability to be sexy ever again. It's a whirlwind of vaginal dryness, bladder leaks, and that unsettling sensation of losing control over our bodies. No wonder we are an insecure mess!

So, what led you to pick up this book? What lit that spark that brought you here? Perhaps it was those sizzling hot flashes that made you wonder if you were secretly auditioning for a sauna commercial.

Well, I am right here with you, and I want to break through stereo-types like never before. Allow me to introduce you to our steadfast companion for this ride: the Full Circle Framework.

Throughout this book, we'll look deeply into:

- **Physical well-being:** We're going to reclaim our bodies and make those hot flashes wish they'd never crossed our path.
- **Emotional resilience:** Prepare to embrace your emotions, ride out those mood swings, and emerge even stronger.
- **Social dynamics:** It's high time we rewrote the script on how society perceives us and how we perceive ourselves.
- **Sexual empowerment:** Rediscover your sensuality and rekindle the flames of desire.
- **Spiritual connection:** Find your inner Zen and reconnect with the spiritual side you never knew existed.

- **Freedom and reinvention:** This is your opportunity to redefine yourself and your purpose.
- **Legacy building:** Leave your mark on the world in a way that's uniquely you.

Now, why should you turn the page? I'll keep it real. I will make you laugh at what we are all going through. Think of this book as your express route to recapturing your vitality, confidence, and zest for life. Picture feeling wanted and acknowledged for your inner and outer beauty, despite society's standards. Imagine rediscovering yourself and seizing back your identity after years of focusing on others.

We've got some seriously inspiring stories of transformation, and who knows? You might even find a few celebrity examples thrown in the mix.

I'm not here to claim guru status, but I've walked and will continue to walk in your shoes, experiencing the same discomfort, insecurity, and loss of control.

So, crack open this book with an open mind and a readiness to challenge everything you believe about menopause. Together, we're going to prove that this is precisely the book we've all wanted and needed. Get ready, ladies, because we're about to embark on an unforgettable, authentic, and empowering adventure through menopause like you've never experienced before!

Chapter 1
Hot Topics, Cold Receptions: Society's Iceberg Approach to Menopause

Former First Lady Michelle Obama knows what's up. She said,

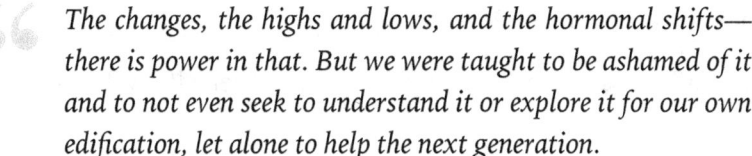 *The changes, the highs and lows, and the hormonal shifts— there is power in that. But we were taught to be ashamed of it and to not even seek to understand it or explore it for our own edification, let alone to help the next generation.*

Ladies, listen up, because we're about to embark on a wild ride through the newly charted territory of menopause. You know, that phase of life that's been shrouded in mystery, whispered about behind closed doors, and referred to as "the change." But let me tell you, it's time to throw those preconceptions out the window and rewrite the script on menopause.

Susan's Story

Susan is in her late 40s and staring down the barrel of menopause like it's a speeding freight train headed straight for her. Anxiety wraps its icy fingers around her as she notices the first telltale signs: the occasional hot flash, a sudden night sweat that turns her bedsheets into a makeshift slip 'n slide—and don't even get her started on the sudden mood swings that seem more reminiscent of her teenage years than her middle-aged ones. Susan is terrified, and she doesn't know where to turn.

For years, she's absorbed the negative societal narrative about menopause. It's been this looming specter of decline, a sort of biological "beginning of the end" for women. She's seen her mother go through it, but it's always been a hushed affair, discussed only behind closed doors and accompanied by furrowed brows and sighs of resignation. Menopause, as far as Susan knows, is just a polite euphemism for a life sentence of hormonal chaos.

But then, one day, Susan has a chance encounter with her friend, Karen, over a cup of coffee. As Susan reluctantly spills her woes about her impending menopausal doom, Karen leans in, her eyes dancing with mischief. "Girl," Karen says with a twinkle in her eye, "you're looking at this all wrong."

Susan raises an eyebrow, intrigued despite herself. "What do you mean?"

Karen leans closer, lowering her voice conspiratorially. "Menopause is like the world's greatest makeover. It's your body's way of saying, 'Hey, I've been through a lot, and now I'm ready to shine like never before. It's time to live for me!'"

Susan blinks, her mind doing somersaults as she contemplates this novel idea. A makeover? Could menopause actually be a glorious new beginning rather than an agonizing end?

At that moment, something clicks inside Susan's brain. She realizes that she doesn't have to be a passive victim of menopause, dreading every symptom and change. She can take charge of her narrative, redefine her own experience, and transform this phase of life into something fabulous.

Chapter 1

As we work through this chapter, we'll look deeper into this newfound perspective. We'll challenge the stereotypes and debunk the myths. Together, we'll emerge from this stronger, more confident women. Get ready because the "menopause makeover" is about to begin, and it's going to be one heck of a ride!

What Society Thinks of Menopause

Menopause—that thing nobody seems to want to talk about but everyone loves to joke about. But guess what? We're changing the perspective on this one!

So, let's dive right in and talk about how the world at large portrays menopause. It's like we're stuck in some bizarre time warp where we're expected to learn how to knit and disappear from the face of the earth. Seriously, who came up with that plan? But hey, we're not having any of that. We're taking charge!

In movies, TV shows, and even medical discussions, menopause is often depicted as the ultimate downslide. You've seen it: Women going through "the change" are portrayed as irritable, depressed, or just plain unhinged. It's like we're expected to turn into these grumpy, gray-haired, sweater-knitting hermits overnight.

And let's not forget those hot flash jokes, mood swing anecdotes, and endless quips about weight gain. Seriously, can we get a new punchline? These stereotypes only perpetuate the negativity surrounding menopause. It's no wonder we hesitate to talk about it seriously when the world insists on making it the butt of every joke.

Even the medical community can sometimes miss the mark. They often zoom in on the clinical aspects of menopause, like potential health risks—think osteoporosis and heart disease. While that is important, it can leave us feeling like we're heading straight for a medical emergency rather than a natural life transition. And don't even get us started on the outdated beliefs!

I will never forget reading a quote from Dr. Robert A. Wilson. "The unpalatable truth must be faced that all post-menopausal women are castrates. Our streets abound with them—walking stiffly in twos and threes, seeing little and observing less. It is not unusual to see an erect man of 75 vigorously striding along a golf course, but never a woman of this age. Now, for the first time in history, women may share the promise of tomorrow as biological equals of men. Thanks to hormone therapy, they can be feminine forever" (Warrick, 1994).

What!? Did this man just compare post-menopausal women to walking zombies? Unfortunately, this was so true at the time. Yeah, that's so outdated, it's almost comical. We're not here to stay locked in some bygone era of thinking. Thanks to modern medicine and a whole lot of common sense, we can absolutely be feminine and fabulous forever, with or without hormones.

But all these portrayals, whether in the media, popular culture, or medical discourse, make one thing clear: Society has us dreading menopause like it's the end of the world. It's time to shift the narrative and realize that menopause isn't about decline, loss, or aging. It's about embracing a new chapter, full of possibilities and laughter—okay, maybe a little sweat, too.

So, my fellow menopausal warriors, let's stop letting these stereotypes and misinformation define our journey. We're aging, not dying, and we're doing it with style and sass!

Common Misconceptions

Let's clear up some of those wild misconceptions that have been floating around for far too long. You know, those myths that make it sound like we're about to embark on a one-way ticket to the land of brain fog and thinning hair. Well, I'm here to tell you that it's not all doom and gloom. In fact, menopause can be a pretty interesting adventure if we embrace it with the right attitude.

Misconception #1: Menopause Means the End of the Road

Oh, boy, have we heard this one before! The idea that menopause is the final stop on the train to Womanhood, and once you're there, it's all downhill. Well, let me set the record straight: Menopause is not the end; it's a new beginning! It's like finishing one book in your life series and eagerly anticipating the sequel. You're not retiring; you're shifting gears.

Misconception #2: Menopause Makes You Invisible

There's this notion that once you hit menopause, you become invisible to the world. Well, I call BS. We are not fading into the background; we are stepping into the spotlight. Menopause is a time to reclaim your identity and let your inner light shine brighter than ever before. You don't need anyone else's validation to feel desirable, sexy, and relevant. You're fabulous, and you know it! We have spent years giving ourselves to motherhood, being a wife, and being an employee—among a hundred other titles. This is our time to give to ourselves!

Misconception #3: Menopause Is All About Decline

Sure, menopause comes with some changes in your body, but it's not all about decline and decay. It's about transformation and growth. Think of it as no longer fitting into a societal shoebox—no longer worrying about what is trending. Your wisdom and experience are your superpowers now. You're not limited by your age; you're empowered by it.

Misconception #4: Goodbye, Intimacy

One of the most common myths is that menopause means waving goodbye to your sex life. Well, let's clear that up right now.

Menopause doesn't mean the end of intimacy; it means redefining what intimacy means to you. It's an opportunity to explore new dimensions of connection with your partner, and with a little creativity, great lube, and open conversation, you can keep the flames of passion burning!

Misconception #5: Menopause Equals Misery

You've probably heard horror stories about the dreaded hot flashes, night sweats, and hormonal mood swings. While these challenges are real, they don't define your entire menopausal experience. Menopause can be a time of self-discovery, personal growth, and even a good laugh at those hot flash moments. It is merely about educating ourselves on how we can best handle what is thrown our way. Did you know bamboo pajamas suck that nightly sweat right up? Remember, laughter is the best medicine!

Let's start tossing these misconceptions out the window and giving menopause a new image—an exciting chapter in our lives. It's a time to reinvent ourselves, rekindle our passions, and redefine what it means to be fabulous at any age.

Why We Need to Talk More About Menopause

I'd like to have a conversation about just that—the power of open dialogue.

You see, for far too long, menopause has been wrapped up in silence and secrecy, like it's some kind of top-secret government operation. Well, news flash, it's not! It's a completely natural and inevitable phase of life.

There used to be a time when we never uttered the word "puberty," and now our children are well-educated about it, as they should be. Do you remember the early days of being pregnant? There were no birthing classes or hospital tours. Fathers were not even in attendance when some of us gave birth. The point is, we have evolved, and so should the conversation around menopause.

The misconceptions and myths about menopause we discussed have been running rampant because we haven't been talking about them. It's like trying to solve a puzzle without all the pieces or trying to cook a gourmet meal with no ingredients—it's a recipe for confusion and stress!

The silence surrounding menopause has led to a whole bunch of misunderstandings, unnecessary anxiety, and stress for women like us who are either approaching or right smack in the middle of it. And let's be honest, nobody needs that kind of drama in their lives!

So, why is open dialogue so important? Well, here are a few reasons that should convince you to break the silence and join the conversation:

- **Reduced stigma:** When we start talking openly about menopause, we're taking a sledgehammer to the walls of stigma. Menopause is not some dirty little secret; it's a part of life, and it's high time we embrace it without shame.
- **Increased support:** Ladies, we all need a little help sometimes, whether it's from healthcare professionals, friends, or family. When we feel comfortable discussing our menopause experiences, we're more likely to seek and receive the support we need. Imagine having a whole squad of people cheering you on through this journey—that's what open dialogue can bring.
- **Understanding better:** Let's face it; ignorance isn't always bliss. When we have open conversations about menopause, we're not only educating ourselves but also those around us. The more we understand what's happening to our bodies, the better equipped we are to deal with it. Knowledge is power, after all!

- **Reframing menopause:** Menopause doesn't have to be a dreaded stage of life. Through open dialogue, we can flip the script and start seeing it as a time of growth, empowerment, and positive transformation. Yes, you heard me right—it can be a time when we shine brighter than ever before!

- **Normalizing the natural:** By chatting openly about menopause, we're helping to normalize this completely natural life stage. We're saying, "Hey, world, this is part of who we are, and we're not hiding it anymore!" And in doing so, we contribute to a broader cultural shift toward a more empowering view of aging and women's health.

Let's break free from the chains of silence and embrace menopause with bright eyes and even wider smiles. Together, we can turn this phase of life into one heck of an adventure, filled with laughter, support, and newfound wisdom.

Menopause: The New Beginning

I know what you're thinking—menopause, ugh, right? It's often been painted as the grand finale, the end of the line, the swan song of our youth. But let's get one thing straight right off the bat—that perspective couldn't be more limiting or inaccurate!

Menopause isn't the end of an era; it's the start of a thrilling new chapter in the book of our lives. So, let's continue to flip the script, shall we?

Picture it like this: You're embarking on a journey, and this isn't just any journey; it's *your* journey. It's a fresh start, a clean slate, and an opportunity to reinvent yourself in ways you may never have imagined. Menopause isn't the closing of a door; it's the opening of a brand-new one, leading to exciting opportunities.

Chapter 1

Now, let's talk about some of these marvelous opportunities that menopause brings to the table. It's time to view it as a renaissance rather than a finale.

First and foremost, think about the freedom! No more monthly periods. Can I get a hallelujah? Say goodbye to tampons, pads, and cramps. It's like a monthly subscription to freedom from that annoying visitor who overstays its welcome.

And speaking of freedom, remember the constant worry about unwanted pregnancies? Poof! Gone. You're free to enjoy intimacy without the lingering anxiety of the "what ifs." Menopause is like a built-in contraceptive—how convenient!

But it's not only about what you're leaving behind; it's also about what you're gaining. Menopause is your time to focus on yourself. Yes, you heard that right. For years, we've been spinning plates—juggling kids, spouses, careers, and countless other responsibilities. Now, it's your time to take center stage.

Menopause is your cue to be unapologetically *you*. It's a time to reflect, grow, and embrace your authentic self. You've spent years being a mother, partner, and professional, but who are you at your core? Menopause is your golden ticket to rediscover yourself, rekindle your passions, and prioritize your dreams.

Let's not forget about the newfound sense of self-confidence and vitality that can come with this phase of life. You are still as vibrant, desirable, and sexy as ever. The mirror may show a few wrinkles and gray hairs, but your inner beauty and charisma are timeless. Society's standards of beauty can take a backseat; you're driving this car now.

Sure, we'll chat about the not-so-glamorous aspects of menopause, too, but we won't dwell on them because they don't define us. These are just temporary inconveniences on our journey to self-discovery and empowerment.

As we embark on this adventure together, remember this: Menopause isn't a full stop; it's a comma, a breath before the next exhilarating chapter. Get ready to embrace this new beginning with a welcoming spirit and a heart full of optimism—because the best is yet to come!

Chapter 1 Challenge: Self-Reflection

I would love to recommend the art of journaling as you make your way through menopause. It gives you a great opportunity to reflect on the times—good, bad, and ugly.

Don't know how to start? Well, here are some journal prompts to help you reflect on your feelings and emotions about your menopause journey:

- **Embracing change:** Write about a recent experience or realization that made you think differently about menopause. How has your perception evolved?
- **Society's influence:** Consider how societal norms and media portray menopause and aging. How have these external influences shaped your own beliefs about this phase of life?
- **Self-image and confidence:** Reflect on how your self-image and confidence have changed as you've aged. What aspects of yourself do you feel most confident about now, and what areas would you like to work on?
- **Desires and aspirations:** Think about what you hope to achieve or experience during and after menopause. Are there any dreams or goals you've put on hold that you're now eager to pursue?
- **Challenges and triumphs:** Recall a challenge related to menopause or aging that you've faced and describe how you overcame it. What did you learn from that experience?

Chapter 1

- **Body positivity:** Write about your relationship with your body and how it has evolved with age. What practices or mindset shifts have helped you maintain a positive body image?
- **Defying stereotypes:** Explore moments when you've defied stereotypes or societal expectations related to aging and menopause. How did it make you feel, and what did you learn from these experiences?

These journal prompts should encourage you to dive deep into your thoughts and emotions surrounding menopause and aging, fostering self-awareness and a more positive outlook on this transformative phase of life.

As we wrap up this chapter, I want you to take a moment and give yourself a well-deserved pat on the back. You've packed your bags and are ready to start this trip to rewrite the story of menopause, and trust me, you're in for one heck of an adventure!

In a world that often portrays menopause as the end of the road, a one-way ticket to the recliner with a blanket and some knitting, we're flipping the script. We're not passengers on a train headed for Grannyville. No, my friends, we're the ones operating this train, and we're taking it to places we've never been before.

We refuse to be defined solely by our age or hormonal fluctuations. We're done with the idea that menopause is a downhill slide into oblivion. Instead, we're embracing it as an opportunity to shine even brighter, to strut our stuff, and to rewrite the rules about what it means to be a vibrant, confident, and sexy woman.

So, as we move forward, let's keep our heads held high, our hearts wide open, and our sense of humor intact. The next chapter will explore the nitty-gritty of the changes we can expect during menopause and how to take care of ourselves along the way. Spoiler alert: It's not just about self-care; it's about self-celebration!

Chapter 2
Redefining Normal Because Normal Is Overrated

Back in the 1800s, Mary Ann Evans was an English novelist, poet, journalist, and translator. Knowing that female writers were not taken seriously, she used the pen name George Eliott to get published and had this to say:

 It's never too late to be what you might have been.

How excellent is that bit of wisdom? Make it your daily mantra. Every day can be the start of something new for you.

Okay, ladies, let's dive headfirst into the menopausal madness, shall we? Buckle up because we're about to tackle the physical changes that make us want to shake our fists at the universe one minute and laugh hysterically the next.

Joanne's Story

Joanne is a badass nurse with 35 years of saving lives under her belt, four kids who've finally left the nest, and a newly minted ex-husband who believes the secret to eternal youth lies in dating women half his age. Joanne is the poster child for selflessness; she's given her life to caring for others, but now it's time to turn that nurturing spirit inward.

Two years ago, as menopause crept in uninvited, Joanne's world got a little topsy-turvy. She thought she had the flu—for six weeks! Waking up soaked through her pajamas? Check. Sweating buckets at work to the point of dizziness? Check. Crying over patient care, usually reserved for private moments, now happening in front of Gertrude's family while discussing her dinner menu of green Jell-O? Triple check.

And then, like many of us, Joanne's inner alarm clock went off, and she blamed it all on stress. She tried everything—lavender, sleep masks, and countless other gadgets that promised relief. The result? Everything annoyed her, and it seemed like she was more tangled in the chaos of menopause than ever.

One day, Joanne found herself sitting in the workplace lunchroom discussing her impending retirement with a coworker she wasn't particularly close to. Tears trickled down her cheeks, and she couldn't control them. When her coworker asked if she was okay, Joanne burst into laughter. She was laughing at herself because she was so far from okay. She had no clue where this emotion was even coming from.

It was at this moment her coworker shared a secret with her. She'd started seeing a hormone specialist. Joanne was initially defensive and accusatory. What was her coworker implying? Was she saying Joanne was broken? It took a few days of soul-searching and confronting the "M" word—menopause—for Joanne to realize something important. She needed to change her perspective. She needed to stop treating menopause like a dirty word or a dark secret and instead embrace it.

Joanne, like all of us, needed to reframe this stage of life. She wanted to find beauty and hope amidst the hot flashes and night sweats. And that, my dear friends, is what this chapter is all about.

We're going to lay it all bare—every awkward chin hair, every hot flash-induced meltdown, and every inexplicable weight gain that's left us befuddled. This chapter isn't here to sugarcoat the struggles; it's here to show how women like Joanne, like you, like me, have faced this rollercoaster with little to no guidance. But it's also here to provide education, hope, and laughter.

So, get ready, because we're about to navigate the wild waters of menopause together. Grab your sense of humor and a glass of wine if you fancy, and let's turn this chapter into a fun, real, and ultimately empowering journey. Menopause may be one hell of a ride, but we're steering this train, and it's going to be epic!

Full-Circle Framework Component #1: Physical Well-Being

Menopause is a bit like the seasons changing, but with some quirky twists. Imagine you're the star of your own reality TV show called *Menopause Makeover*.

In this show, your body is the set, and each season symbolizes a different stage of menopause:

Spring—Perimenopause

This is when your body starts dropping hints that change is coming, like Mother Nature teasing you with a few warm days before spring officially arrives. Your hormones begin to play pranks on you, and it's like your body's way of saying, "Get ready for some surprises!" This is like the appetizer to the main course of menopause. It typically starts in your 40s but can sneak up on you as early as your 30s. Think of it as your body's way of saying, "Hey, remember all those sleepless nights you had with a crying baby? Well, here are some sleepless nights with hot flashes as a bonus!"

Summer—Menopause

The heat is on, baby! It's like the sweltering days of summer, where you're sweating buckets and dealing with hot flashes that make you feel like you're in the Sahara Desert. Just like a summer vacation, there are moments of excitement and moments where you wish you were somewhere cooler. This is the main event! Typically, you can expect this around age 51. But remember, Mother Nature has a quirky sense of humor, and she might show up early or late—just like your favorite tardy friend who always has an excuse. This is when Aunt Flo officially waves the white flag and moves to Greece, and you haven't seen her for at least 12 consecutive months. It's like your uterus decided to take an extended vacation without you. And to celebrate this milestone, it throws a party with symptoms like hot flashes, mood swings, and insomnia, just for fun. How long does all this fun last? I knew you were going to ask. You can expect this to last, on average, four years. Read that again.

Fall—Post-Menopause

Ah, the golden years. This is like the calm after the storm, when the leaves start to change color. Your hormones are settling down, and you're enjoying a more peaceful time. It's like a crisp autumn day after a scorching summer, where you can finally relax and sip on your pumpkin spice latte. This is like the after-party but without the cocktails. Once you've hit the one-year mark without a period, you're officially postmenopausal. Your hormones start to settle down, but don't expect them to go quietly into the night. They might just leave you with a few souvenirs, like vaginal dryness or hair loss. Thanks, hormones!

Chapter 2

Winter—Wisdom Years

This is when you've fully embraced the wisdom that comes with age. You've survived the ups and downs of menopause and can now share your hilarious stories and sage advice with others. It's like the serene beauty of a winter landscape, where you've come out on the other side stronger and wiser. For the love of all things hormonal, *please* share all you have learned. We do not talk enough about this, and we want to try and educate those beautiful women coming up behind us.

So, menopause is like starring in your own reality show where your body goes through different seasons, each with its own set of surprises and challenges. And just like any good reality show, there are plenty of laughs, drama, and memorable moments along the way.

But why, oh why, does menopause happen? Well, it's like this: Your ovaries decide they've had enough of producing eggs and running the hormonal roller coaster, and they decide to throw in the towel. Your estrogen, progesterone, and testosterone levels go off the rails, and you end up feeling like you're in a never-ending nightmare.

Speaking of hormones, let's get to know our hormone squad a little better (*Menopause Hormones – What Are They and How Do They Change?* 2020):

- **Estrogen:** the diva of hormones, and there are three types! Estradiol, estrone, and estriol They're like the Spice Girls of your body, and they love to light things up by causing mood swings and hot flashes.
- **Progesterone:** the peacekeeper hormone. It tries to calm down the estrogen drama, but sometimes it just gives up and joins the party.

- **Testosterone:** Yep, we ladies have it, too, just in smaller amounts. Testosterone is like your inner rock star; it's responsible for your sex drive and muscle mass. But during menopause, it can take a nosedive and leave you feeling like a deflated balloon.

So there you have it—a short but sweet crash course on menopause. It's like going through puberty all over again, but with the added bonus of adulting responsibilities. Remember, we're in this together, and we're taking back control. Menopause is just another chapter in our fabulous lives, and we're going to tackle it with humor, resilience, and a whole lot of chin-hair jokes. Stay tuned for more adventures in the world of menopause, my brave friends!

What Is Happening to My Body?

If you have ever woken up one day and thought, *What on earth is actually happening to my body?* You are in the right place! Once upon a time, it was thought that menopause made us all "crazy," and as the years passed, the entire focus was around hot flashes. It is time to explore all of the physical changes that come along with the menopausal journey (*Top 10 Symptoms of Low Estrogen*, 2019):

- **Cold flushes:** Imagine going from feeling like a human torch one moment to an ice cube the next. That's menopause for you. Cold flushes, the lesser-known sibling of hot flashes, will have you reaching for that sweater and then ripping it off in record time. Cause? Estrogen levels are going bonkers!
- **Tingling in extremities:** Ever get that weird sensation in your hands and feet, like they've fallen asleep without your permission? Welcome to the tingling extremities club. It's like your body's way of reminding you that it's the boss,

and it's got some surprises in store. Cause? Yep, you guessed it: low estrogen!

- **Fatigue:** Ah, the uninvited guest that is fatigue, also caused by messed up estrogen levels. It might seem like you've run a marathon after a leisurely stroll to the mailbox. Menopause fatigue can zap your energy faster than your kids empty the fridge.

- **Decreased libido:** Remember when your libido was on fire? Well, now it's more like a flickering candle. Menopause can take a toll on your desire, but fear not; we've got tricks up our sleeves to reignite that flame.

- **Thinning hair:** Say hello to your hairbrush and wave goodbye to your once-luscious locks. Thinning hair (everywhere 😉) can be frustrating, but it's all part of the menopausal package. Those plummeting estrogen levels do a number on us. On the plus side, no more shaving!

- **Burning mouth, missed periods, vertigo, anxiety, vaginal dryness, changes in spatial awareness, depression:** Yeah, you read that right, and that's not even the whole list! Menopause and our crazy hormone levels can throw all kinds of curveballs our way. Your mouth might feel like it's on fire, periods might become as elusive as a unicorn, and you could get dizzy spells that make you question your sense of direction. It's like a carnival of symptoms!

- **Itchy skin, tinnitus, brittle nails, changes in taste, breast tenderness, changes in body odor:** And the hits just keep coming! Feeling like something's crawling on your skin when there's nothing there? Check. Hearing phantom sounds in your ears? Check. Nails as brittle as your favorite snack? Check. Menopause certainly keeps you guessing.

While these symptoms may sound like a never-ending list of woes, remember that menopause is a deeply personal journey. Each of us is a unique snowflake, and our menopausal experiences vary like snowflakes themselves. Some might get the whole smorgasbord of symptoms, while others may breeze through with hardly a hiccup. Remember, we don't hate those women; we just wish we were them!

So, as you navigate these physical changes, remember to keep your sense of humor intact. Menopause may throw some surprises your way, but you've got the power to laugh, learn, and saunter through this wild life with delight. After all, we're not taking menopause as the end of the line; we're reclaiming our lives and seizing the day with a smile, even if it's a slightly sweaty one!

Wine, Chocolate, and Yoga Pants: Surviving Menopause With Healthy Living

It's now time to tackle the topic of a healthy lifestyle during menopause with a big dose of humor and camaraderie.

First off, let me lay it out for you: Menopause is like the surprise party you never asked to be invited to. It crashes into your life with exhaustion, dizziness, and the sudden urge to throw your bathroom scale out the window (because who needs that kind of negativity?). But the good news is that you have more control over this transition than you might think.

Did you know that the daily decisions you make, from the foods you eat to the amount of sleep you get, can directly affect the intensity and occurrence of menopausal symptoms? I can confess: I had *no* clue.

Food: Eat the Damn Cake

Now, let's talk about food. I know! We've all had our fair share of diets, from Atkins to juice cleanses. But here's the deal: We're not here to hop on the latest diet trend and count every calorie like it's our second job. We have earned this time to enjoy the skin we are in. Menopause is simply a time when our bodies need some extra love and attention.

So, instead of stressing about what you can't eat, focus on what you can. It's all about balance. Yes, you can have that cake, just maybe not for breakfast, lunch, *and* dinner. Throw in some greens and lots of protein. Nourish your body with foods that make you feel good, both inside and out. Embrace those comfort foods now more than ever and balance them out with plenty of fruits, veggies, proteins, and whole grains. There's a lot of new, interesting research on intermittent fasting. It may not be so much *what* you eat as *when* you eat. Check it out.

Remember, food is not the enemy. It's your ally in this menopausal journey. Life is short—eat the damn cake!

Exercise: Move It, Groove It

Now, let's talk about exercise. I know the thought of hitting the gym might be about as appealing as a root canal right now. But here's the secret: You don't have to go all-out in those kickboxing classes unless that's your jam. What's important is that you move your body in a way that feels good for you.

Whether it's a nice walk in the park with the grandkids, getting around the block with the fur baby, or a dance party in your living room, the key is to love it. Exercise is not just about losing weight; it's about clearing out those mental cobwebs and boosting those mood-lifting endorphins.

So, here's your mission, should you choose to accept it: Find an activity that brings you joy. It could be yoga, swimming, hiking, or even one of those new pole dancing classes—now that's a workout! Because, honestly, nobody is watching, and even if they are, who cares? You're worth the energy and effort it takes to move your beautiful, menopausal body.

Let's not make menopause a time of restriction and deprivation. It's a time to celebrate our bodies, enjoy delicious food, and move in ways that make us happy. We're in this together, and with a bit of humor, a piece of cake, and a sprinkle of movement, we can navigate this journey with style, grace, and a whole lot of laughter.

Bring On the Wrinkles and Wisdom

Ladies, let's dive headfirst into the deep end of menopause and tackle the notion of aging gracefully. I know what you're thinking. *Aging gracefully? I can't even gracefully open a pickle jar anymore!* But let's get one thing straight: Aging gracefully isn't about holding on to your 20s like a desperate lifeline. No, it's about embracing the glorious mess that is menopause with a sense of humor, a touch of sass, and a whole lot of self-love.

You see, society bombards us with anti-aging products and ideals that make us feel like we're in a never-ending battle against time. We're told that aging means losing our vitality, becoming a victim of illness, and falling behind in the race to keep up with the world. Let's take a look at a few of those now:

- **"Erase wrinkles instantly!"**: These ads often show impossibly flawless models with not a wrinkle in sight, implying that wrinkles are something to be ashamed of. Do they show a model of our age using this product with amazing results? No. We aren't meant to travel back in time, people.

- **"Turn back the clock!"**: These messages suggest that aging is undesirable and that we should strive to look and feel younger, reinforcing the idea that getting older is something to fear.
- **"Youth in a bottle!"**: Promising to bottle up the fountain of youth, these ads create unrealistic expectations, making women feel like they're missing out if they don't use these products.
- **"Banish gray hair!"**: These ads promote the idea that gray hair is unacceptable or unattractive, pushing women to dye their hair to hide their natural aging process.
- **"Look 10 years younger!"**: These ads can create a sense of inadequacy by suggesting that looking your actual age is somehow undesirable or inferior.
- **"Stay forever young!"**: Promoting the idea that youthfulness is the ultimate goal, these ads can make women feel like they're failing if they don't achieve eternal youth.
- **"The secret to ageless beauty!"**: These messages often promise a "secret" to staying young, creating a sense of exclusion for those who don't have access to the supposed secret.
- **"Rediscover your lost youth!"**: These ads can make women feel like they've lost something valuable as they age, rather than recognizing the wisdom and experience that comes with it.
- **"Don't let aging hold you back!"**: This implies that aging is a limitation or barrier rather than a natural part of life with its own unique beauty and opportunities.

You won't believe this, but in 2021, the anti-aging market was raking in a jaw-dropping 62.6 billion U.S. dollars worldwide! Billion—with a "B." And guess what? It's not slowing down anytime soon. Experts predict that it's going to keep growing at a crazy rate of nearly seven percent every year from 2022 to 2027 (*Size of the Anti-Aging Market Worldwide 2018–2023*, 2018).

I mean, seriously, it's like the whole world is trying to sell us the idea that aging is a crime we need to prevent at all costs. But we know better, right? We're here to embrace the fabulous journey of aging gracefully, not just pour our hard-earned money into anti-aging products to feel accepted by society. And let's take a moment to be real. We have all, at one time or another, spent our money on some of these products. Have you ever found a miracle in a bottle? Exactly. So, let's start putting our money into things we actually benefit from, like pole dancing classes and new trail runners!

Aging gracefully means looking in the mirror, beautiful wrinkles and all, and saying, "You're more fabulous than ever." It's about appreciating the life you have lived and acknowledging that your body is getting better with age, getting better with acceptance. Sure, things might not be as perky as they used to be, but you've seen more, experienced more, and earned every laugh line and wrinkle.

Now, let's talk about self-compassion. It's not just some feel-good advice from a motivational poster. Research has shown that women with high levels of self-compassion experience those pesky hot flashes, too. But those flashes bother them much less. Why? Because they've got a compassionate inner cheerleader saying, "It's okay, hot stuff, this too shall pass (Haak, 2014)."

Self-compassion isn't about pretending that mood swings and night sweats are your new BFFs. No, it's about treating yourself with the same kindness, concern, and understanding that you'd offer to your best friend going through the same thing.

Let's revisit our good friend Joanne. She was so hard on herself throughout her entire menopause journey. At each crossroads, she belittled herself, bought into all the anti-aging products, and revisited every crash diet. Six months later, her best friend, Diane, would come to her in tears. It would seem the menopause fairy had started to pay her a visit.

Joanne found herself being this solid sounding board to her friend. She offered great advice, reminding Diane that this was all part of being a strong woman. She told Diane some great tricks and tips she had learned so far. They started doing weekly walks together to get their bodies moving. It was during one of these walks that Diane noticed just how hard Joanne was on herself. She stopped them both, looked Joanne in the eye, and said softly, "You should speak to yourself the same way you speak to me."

From that point on, Joanne was able to see things from a whole new perspective. Her friend was right. She did deserve compassion and self-love. There was no reason she shouldn't be engaging in this to get through this season of life.

You, too, should remember this while recognizing that these changes in your body are as normal as the changing seasons and don't make you any less fabulous.

So, when you catch a glimpse of your reflection in the midst of a hot flash-induced glow or poking that fluffy belly for the umpteenth time, remember this: You're aging gracefully, my friend.

Chapter 2 Challenge: Expressing Gratitude

Okay, ladies, let's take a moment to give our bodies a big, virtual high-five. We've just danced our way through a chapter full of the wild and wacky adventures of menopause, and now it's time for some well-deserved gratitude.

So, grab a cup or glass of your favorite beverage, a slice of chocolate cake, put on your comfiest pair of pajamas, and settle into a cozy chair. Let's show some love to the incredible vessel that is our body.

Complete this statement: "Today, I am grateful for my body because...

- **It's a survivor:** Our bodies have been through some serious changes during menopause, but guess what? They've made it this far! From teenage acne to those night sweats that rival Niagara Falls, our bodies have weathered every storm and kept us going. So, today, let's appreciate the resilience that our bodies have shown.
- **It's a hug magnet:** Who doesn't love a good hug? Our bodies allow us to feel the warmth and comfort of a loving embrace, whether it's from your kids, your partner, or your furry friend. Hugs are like mini-vacations for the soul, and we owe it all to our sense of touch.
- **It's a superhero:** Remember those days when you could carry a week's worth of groceries in one trip without breaking a sweat? Well, even though we might not be lifting as effortlessly now, our bodies still do amazing things. They heal wounds, digest food, and keep everything ticking along. Our bodies are like the unsung superheroes of the daily grind.
- **It's a sensation machine:** Our bodies are equipped with an intricate network of nerves that allow us to experience the world in all its glory. From the taste of our favorite sweet treat to the feel of a cool breeze on our skin, our bodies are our ticket to the sensory rollercoaster of life.
- **It's a journey, buddy:** Through all the ups and downs of life, our bodies have been right there with us. They've carried us through joy, sorrow, adventure, and laughter. Our bodies are our trusty companions on this crazy ride called life.

Chapter 2

Remember, ladies, our bodies are pretty darn amazing, and they've served us well through thick and thin. So, let's raise a glass to these fantastic vessels that have brought us this far. Gratitude isn't just about appreciating the good; it's about embracing every part of ourselves because it's our bodies that carry us forward into this exciting new phase of life.

We are warriors, and warriors don't back down from a challenge. We might feel like our bodies are betraying us at times, but we're here to remind ourselves that we're still the fierce, funny, and fabulous individuals we've always been. Menopause might make us doubt ourselves from time to time, but we're ready to get educated and conquer this.

Now, let's take a deep breath and get ready for the next part of our journey: the emotional struggles we face in menopause. Just like those physical symptoms, this chapter is going to be intense and real. But remember, we've got each other, and together, we can laugh, cry, and tackle anything that comes our way. So, grab your favorite snacks, pour yourself a glass of something delicious (whether it's a green smoothie or a glass of wine—I won't judge), and let's dive into the emotional world that is menopause.

Chapter 3
Tears, Cheers, and Emotional Gears

According to investigative reporter Lisa Jey Davis,

> *You can do this—this thing, where your body will cease to produce hormones and your skin, hair, muscles and bones ... basically every part of you will notice, go into withdrawals, and stage a coup. Be prepared for this mentally, and you'll own this 'thing.'*

It's a typical morning, and you're standing in your kitchen, desperately trying to salvage your burned breakfast. The tears are welling up in your eyes as you contemplate the tragedy that is your charred toast. In your hormonal haze, it seems like the end of the world, and you can't help but cry over something as trivial as toast.

Fast forward to the office, where you find yourself inexplicably irritated during a meeting because someone devoured all the donuts. You're fuming, and your colleagues exchange concerned glances, wondering if you've gone mad. You wonder, *What is wrong with me? They're just donuts!*

By the time evening rolls around, you're yawning your way through the grocery store, glaring at anyone who dares try to cut you off in the aisles. *What ever happened to the person I used to be? The one who would offer to reach the box off the top shelf for someone?* You drive home exhausted, sweat pouring down your back. You think *I'll just get to bed early and get some sleep!* And then "she" shows up—the insomnia fairy. Get some rest? Feel better tomorrow? "Think again," says Menopause.

Sound familiar? If you've been through menopause or are in the midst of it, you probably know exactly what I'm talking about. The emotional turbulence that accompanies this phase can make you feel like you're living in a never-ending sitcom. What I didn't know, and you may not either, is that this is all perfectly normal and expected.

Kim's Story

For the past 35 years, Kim has been the undisputed champion of family Christmas dinner. Since becoming a mother herself, she has taken the reins of this cherished tradition with enthusiasm and love. Every holiday season, her children would playfully ask if she was ready to pass the torch, and every year, her answer was a resounding, "No way!" She took pride in meticulously coordinating everything, from matching placemats to stockings and decorations. Her holiday recipes were a well-guarded treasure, passed down through generations.

However, this year was different. Kim has been experiencing some weird changes in her body. Nights were filled with sweating, dizziness, and unrelenting exhaustion, and sleep had become a luxury. Her mother had never shared a word about menopause, and the few tidbits her friends offered always revolved around humorous tales of chin hairs multiplying like rabbits. The focus had always

Chapter 3

been on the physical symptoms, leaving Kim feeling lost in a sea of unfamiliar emotions.

As the big day of Christmas dinner arrived, Kim had only managed a meager three hours of sleep the night before. The thought of wearing her favorite holiday sweater and apron was quickly dashed, as she'd already melted through her makeup. Instead of cheerful carols filling the air, the family found a frazzled Kim in the kitchen, sporting shorts and a tank top, her hair piled high atop her head. No chipper mother was greeting them with eggnog this time. She was flushed, tears welling up in her eyes.

The grandkids were met with a different grandma than they remembered. She was quick to snap at them, and a cloud of depression seemed to hang over the festivities. The breaking point came when Kim realized her stuffing was dry and the gravy was lumpy. She started ripping down decorations, exclaiming, "Why even bother celebrating?" Her sobbing escalated, leaving her children frozen and unsure of how to respond.

Amidst the chaos, her oldest daughter stepped forward. She knew this was more than just a holiday hiccup. She joined her mother in the bathroom, sitting with her on the floor, offering comforting words and a shoulder to lean on. They decided to order pizza and allow this Christmas be whatever it needed to be, with no pressure to meet past expectations.

Together, they crafted a plan. The next day, they would call the doctor to discuss Kim's symptoms and reach out to her therapist for support. Her daughter reassured her that she would be there every step of the way, helping her figure out this world of menopause, both physically and emotionally.

With the love and support of her family, Kim started to educate herself about the emotional upheaval that menopause can bring.

Nobody talks about this aspect of menopause, and it desperately needs to change. The terrifying whirlwind of emotions that can accompany this life stage catches many women off guard. Kim realized that being prepared and knowing what to do is the key to finding balance and rediscovering herself amid the turbulence of menopause.

In this chapter, we'll share the tips and tools you need to stay afloat during these stormy emotional seas. You'll discover that menopause, despite its chaos, has a silver lining. It's an opportunity for increased self-awareness and emotional strength that you never thought possible.

With newfound perspective and these essential tools, you'll learn not only to embrace your emotions but also to take back control of your life. So, grab your sense of humor, because we're about to dive into the hilarious, relatable, and occasionally messy world of menopause emotions. Together, we'll come out on the other side as stronger, more resilient women who know how to ride the emotional rollercoaster like pros.

Full-Circle Framework Component #2: Emotional Resilience

Let's talk about something we all go through but rarely discuss openly: the absolutely immense range of emotions that can come with menopause and our fluctuating hormones. Grab a comfy seat because we're diving deep into the emotional journey of "the change."

First things first, let's get this straight: You are *not* going crazy. It's not about being "cranky" or "moody." It's about being human and managing a significant life transition. Menopause is a literal decrease in our bodies' hormones, which will cause our emotions to become imbalanced, and it's perfectly okay to feel all of them.

Mood swings? Oh, yes, they're real. One minute you're laughing at a puppy video, and the next, you're in tears because you can't find your keys. It's like emotional whiplash. You may not like it, but this is normal! Your hormones are doing the cha-cha, and your body is adjusting. Give yourself permission to feel these swings without judgment. This too shall pass!

Anxiety may also rear its head during menopause. You might find yourself worrying about everything, from whether you can retire comfortably to wondering if you left the oven on. Again, this is not a sign of weakness—it's a response to the physical and emotional changes happening inside you. Take a few deep breaths and remind yourself that it's okay not to have all the answers. Take it one day at a time.

The fear of losing control is a big one. This one was and still is especially hard for me. Suddenly, it feels like your irregular hormones are driving the train, and you're just along for the ride. It's understandable to be uncomfortable and even angry here. I am an admitted control freak. I like to know the plan before there is even a plan. So, when my body and brain decide to "change things up" just for the fun of it, I am not okay. It can set me back emotionally. I don't like feeling out of control. I have had to lean into some of the strategies in this chapter daily to find my peace with this. One thing that helps me is knowing that I still have control over my choices, how I react, and how I approach this time in my life.

Feeling like you've lost your "former self" or sadness about the passage of time is another common emotional challenge. It's natural to reminisce about your younger years and wonder where the time went. Who wouldn't, right? With all that social media and advertising thrown at us, why wouldn't we always be thinking the best years are behind us? I say enough! Your wisdom and strength have grown with age, and that's something to celebrate.

And let's not forget about rage. Your haywire hormones might make you want to snap over the smallest things. But instead of suppressing it, own your anger and use it as fuel for positive change. We are conditioned to believe that anger is negative, but it is a valid emotion, and we should acknowledge it. It is unhealthy to smother it. Maybe it's time to stand up for what you believe in or set some boundaries in your life.

Remember, it's okay to seek support during this time. Share your feelings with a trusted friend, therapist, or support group. And please, be gentle with yourself. You deserve kindness and compassion as you navigate this journey.

Menopause is not the end; it's a brand-spanking new beginning. Embrace the emotional ups and downs as part of your beautiful, complex self. You are strong, you are resilient, and you are still the incredible person you've always been.

What to Do With All These Feelings

You deserve all the strategies in the world to navigate these complex feelings because, well, you're a badass, and menopause is simply another adventure in this crazy thing we call life.

- **Embrace the meltdown:** Let's start by acknowledging that it's okay to have a meltdown. Have you ever looked at a toddler throwing an all-out tantrum and thought, *I wish I could do that right now?* You know, just throw yourself on the ground and let it all out! I wanted to do this just yesterday, right in the middle of the grocery store. Yet, society would frown, alas! A good meltdown is like hitting the reset button on your emotions. So, grab your favorite tearjerker movie and a box of tissues and let it all out. Or, find your nearest smash class. If you haven't heard of this, it is a safe space where you can go—goggles and protective gear provided—and smash things! It is a great way to get out all that pent-up anxiety, anger, and hostility!

- **Find your people:** Menopause can make you feel like you're on a deserted island, but you're not alone. Reach out to your girlfriends who've been there, done that, and bought the T-shirt. Share your stories, laugh about the absurdity of it all, and remind each other that you're still fabulous. Please have some real conversations while you're together. Talk about the deep stuff and how you are managing. You would be surprised at how much relief you will all get, and you just might pick up some tools from one another.
- **Laugh it off:** Laughter is the best medicine, they say, and for good reason. Find humor in the madness of menopause. Did you accidentally put your keys in the fridge? Did you start a conversation with your dog, thinking it was your partner? It happens to the best of us. Share your funny moments with friends and turn those "senior moments" into legendary tales.
- **Talk to someone:** If you find that your emotions are getting the best of you, don't hesitate to seek professional help. Therapy can provide you with tools and strategies to manage. There's no shame in asking for a helping hand, and it is always fantastic to have someone to unload on.
- **Find what makes you smile:** Remember all those things you used to love before life got in the way? Now is the perfect time to revisit them. Whether it's painting, dancing, cooking, or learning a new skill, reignite your passions and watch your confidence soar.
- **Talk to your partner:** Your partner may not fully understand what you're going through, but open communication is key. Share your feelings, needs, and desires. Let them be your rock and remind you of the strong, sexy woman you are. I want to emphasize this one, and I have a story to share. As menopause started in my life, I often joked about my symptoms because I use humor

when I am uncomfortable. Well, naturally, as time went on and a hot flash would begin, my husband would joke. Internally, I would seethe. *How dare he?* I thought. But why wouldn't he? I taught him that this behavior was okay. After a few months, I sat him down and educated him. I explained what was happening to my body and how it all made me feel. I told him that when he made light of it, I felt he didn't care. It changed how we interacted for the better. Do not be afraid to have these conversations with your partner. It could make the difference between them bringing you an ice pack and you smothering them with a pillow while they sleep.

- **Empower yourself:** Menopause is not the end; it's a new beginning. Embrace this stage of life with all the wisdom and grace you've acquired over the years. Reject the notion that growing older is a bad thing. You are a force to be reckoned with, and the best is yet to come. If you don't feel this way yet, find ways to continue to learn, lean into what you are good at, and explore new and exciting adventures.

- **Celebrate your sexy:** Listen, real talk here. We all know we once had a drawer filled with silky and sexy items that took far too long to put on. We learned throughout the years that we would have kids, pets, and snacks in our beds. Times have changed, and that bed may have you and a partner or just you in it. The question is: What are you going to do about it? Your sex life is on the verge of wonderful things yet again. You no longer have to worry about pregnancy, menstrual cramps, periods, or figuring out how to get that leg above your head—you get the picture here. It is not time to close up shop. Yes, vaginal dryness is here to stay, but lube can make you forget all about it. At this age, you may be blessed with not giving a crap about societal standards regarding body image. That is a huge plus in the bedroom. Own your beautiful body.

Own your sexual intimacy. Pop the top off that lube and enjoy these years. I am a woman in menopause, and I am a woman your age, so I *know* you have earned it!

Meditation

Let's talk about meditation, the secret weapon in our arsenal for riding this emotional wave of menopause. It can help us maintain our sanity and feel more like our vibrant, confident selves.

Picture this: You're lying in bed at night, and the world seems to be conspiring against you with night sweats and racing thoughts. Enter bedtime meditation! It's like a soothing lullaby for your frazzled brain. Close your eyes and take a deep breath. Let's dive into some meditation practices tailored for our menopausal journey.

- **Body scan meditation:** Think of this as a spa day for your mind. Start from the tip of your toes and work your way up, scanning your body for any areas of tension or discomfort. Menopause can bring all sorts of aches and pains, and this meditation helps you release them one by one. Feel the stress melt away as you focus on each body part. Bonus points if you imagine sending warmth and relaxation to those hormonal hotspots!
- **Sensory grounding:** We all have moments when we feel like we're losing control during menopause. Sensory grounding is your ticket to getting back in touch with reality. Find a quiet spot, close your eyes, and take a few deep breaths. Now, pay attention to your senses. What do you hear, smell, taste, and feel in this moment? Grounding yourself in the present can help you regain a sense of control when the hormonal rollercoaster gets bumpy.
- **Loving-kindness meditation:** Menopause can mess with our self-esteem, making us feel less confident and less attractive. This is where loving-kindness meditation

swoops in to save the day. Sit comfortably, close your eyes, and start by sending love and positive vibes to yourself. Imagine wrapping yourself in a warm, cozy blanket of self-compassion. Then, extend that love to others in your life. Remember, you're freaking fabulous, and menopause doesn't define your worth.

- **Bedtime meditation:** Sleep disturbances during menopause can make us feel like zombies during the day. A bedtime meditation ritual can make all the difference. Find a comfortable position in bed, close your eyes, and start focusing on your breath. Breathe in calm and serenity, and exhale stress and worries. Let go of the day's challenges and embrace the promise of a new morning.

Regular meditation isn't a magic potion for all menopausal symptoms, but it can help you find some much-needed calm in the storm. It's your personal escape from the madness, an opportunity to connect with your inner wisdom, and a way to boost your confidence.

Journaling

Grab a notebook and a fancy pen—because who doesn't love fancy pens?—and let's explore the world of emotional journaling.

Let's start by asking ourselves why we should even bother with journaling during menopause. Well, it's like having a private chat with your future self. Writing down your feelings and experiences can be incredibly cathartic and therapeutic. So, how does emotional journaling help, exactly?

Journaling allows you to process your feelings, whether it's frustration, sadness, or even joy. It's like a safe space for your emotions. Even in those times when you don't understand what or why you are feeling them, just getting them out onto the paper can be helpful. It's a mental and emotional purging, if you will.

Chapter 3

Your body is going through some serious changes, and it can be a lot to handle. Writing about your physical and emotional symptoms can help you track patterns and gain insights into what triggers them. It's like being your own detective!

Menopause is a journey of self-discovery. It's a time to reconnect with who you are beyond the roles you've played as a parent, spouse, or career person. Journaling can help you explore your inner thoughts, desires, and dreams. You might even surprise yourself with what you find.

Now, let's get practical with some emotional journaling techniques:

- **Stream of consciousness writing:** Imagine you're chatting with your best friend. Write without judgment or editing. Let your thoughts flow freely onto the paper. Don't worry about grammar or spelling—just let it all out.
- **Gratitude journaling:** Amidst the chaos of menopause, there are moments of beauty and joy. Write down three things you're grateful for every day. It could be as simple as a cup of your favorite tea or taking off that bra at the end of the day. Gratitude helps shift your focus from what's challenging to what's wonderful in your life.
- **Letters to yourself:** Write a letter to your younger self or your future self. What advice would you give? What do you want to remember? It's a beautiful way to connect with different phases of your life and offer yourself compassion and encouragement.
- **Mood tracking:** Create a daily mood chart. Rate your mood on a scale from 1 to 10, and jot down what might have influenced it. Over time, you can spot patterns and identify what lifts you up or brings you down. This is also a great way to set boundaries around what may bring negativity into your life.

- **Creative expression:** Don't limit yourself to just words. Draw, doodle, paint, or use stickers in your journal. Sometimes, expressing your emotions through art can be incredibly freeing.

Remember, there's no right or wrong way to journal. It's your journey, so make it your own. And, hey, if you find yourself laughing at your entries, that's a win!

Breathing Exercises

Let's look into something that can really help you with the ups and downs of the emotional side of menopause: breathing exercises. Yep, you read that right; we're going to give those breaths a makeover that'll make you feel like a goddess in the midst of it all.

- **The cool, calm breath:** You know that feeling when you're about to blow your top because you're suddenly sweating buckets and feeling all sorts of frazzled? Well, this one's for you. The cool, calm breath is all about finding your inner Zen. Take a deep breath in for a count of four, hold it for seven, and then release it slowly over eight counts. It's like your personal air-conditioning for those hot flashes!
- **The hot flush wave:** Picture yourself riding a wave of warmth, and as you inhale deeply through your nose, imagine you're catching that wave at its peak. Then, exhale through your mouth, letting go of the heat as the wave gently carries it away, bringing cool refreshment in its wake. Feel the soothing rhythm of each breath, mirroring the gentle rise and fall of the ocean, leaving you grounded and renewed in the tranquil aftermath of this mindful journey.
- **Straw breath:** Remember how much fun you had sipping your favorite drinks through a straw when you were a kid? Well, this breath is just as delightful! Grab an imaginary

straw and take a slow, smooth inhale through it. Feel the cool air filling you up, and then exhale naturally. It's like sipping on serenity and exhaling stress.

- **Bumblebee breath:** This one's all about making a little noise—a fun, therapeutic noise. Close your eyes, take a deep breath in, and as you exhale, hum like a contented bumblebee. Feel the vibration and let it massage your stress away.

Self-Care

Self-care is important. It is vital. It is critical. There, I said it, and I am going to keep saying it. We do not give ourselves nearly enough attention during menopause, and we need to start.

I don't want you to just read the self-care ideas below; I want you to try them on and see which ones work for you. Then, use them—and use them often. This will have you feeling like the fabulous, vibrant woman you truly are:

- **Get lost in a book:** Remember those times when you couldn't put a good book down? Well, it's time to rediscover that joy. Immerse yourself in novels, magazines, or maybe even some graphic novels—whatever floats your literary boat. It's a fantastic way to escape reality for a while and let your imagination run wild.
- **Try nature's therapy:** Mother Nature is your free therapist, available 24-7. Take walks in the park, explore hiking trails, or just lounge in your backyard, soaking up some sunshine. The great outdoors and all that greenery can work wonders for your mood and overall well-being.
- **Do what you love:** Remember those hobbies you used to adore or always wanted to try? Well, now's your time to shine! Try painting, cooking classes, dancing, or even

picking up a new instrument, like the ukulele. Pursuing your passions can be incredibly fulfilling.

- **Utilize meditation and mindfulness:** Menopause's hormonal upheaval is overwhelming at times, no doubt. That's where meditation and mindfulness step in as your trusty sidekicks. They'll help you stay centered, calm, and focused, no matter what hormonal whirlwind is blowing your way.

- **Do yoga and exercise:** Exercise isn't only a mood booster; it's also a stress reliever. Give yoga a try. It combines physical activity with mindfulness. You don't need to twist yourself into a pretzel; a few simple stretches can work wonders.

- **Hang out with your people:** Round up your besties and have a girls' night out! Laughter is genuinely the best medicine, and sharing stories with friends who are likely experiencing similar adventures can be incredibly therapeutic.

- **Pamper yourself:** Don't forget to treat yourself from time to time. Whether it's a relaxing massage or spa day or simply indulging in a luxurious bath with your favorite scented candles and a good book, pampering yourself is a must.

Now, let's look at the big picture. Menopause isn't just about managing the emotional ride; it's about embracing this new chapter of your life. It's an opportunity to develop new coping strategies and handle stress and anxiety like a pro.

Your emotional strength is like fine wine, getting better with age. This is your time to shine, rediscover yourself, and reclaim your identity and sense of purpose. And guess what? You're more desirable, sexy, confident, and relevant than ever.

Chapter 3 Challenge: Who Are You?

Now, let's talk about expressing those emotions and embracing your inner artist. Menopause is a time of change, and change can be hard. However, it can also be incredibly liberating and inspiring. So, here are some creative ideas to help you get through those emotions and rediscover the beautiful, vibrant you:

- **Create art:** Whether you're an aspiring Picasso or a total novice, grab some paintbrushes or colored pencils and let your emotions flow onto the canvas. Paint a picture that represents your experience with menopause so far. It could be an abstract or a vivid representation of your journey.
- **Visualize your future:** Imagine how you want to feel after navigating menopause. Draw or paint a vision of the confident, empowered woman you aspire to be. This is your opportunity to set your own standards of beauty and vitality.
- **Write your triumphs:** Pick up a journal or open a fresh document on your computer and jot down a moment during your menopause journey when you felt particularly strong or empowered. Reflecting on these moments can boost your self-esteem and remind you of your resilience.
- **Dance:** Choose a song that resonates with how you're feeling right now, whether it's fierce, joyful, or introspective. Crank up the volume and let your body move to the music in any way that feels natural. Dancing is a fantastic way to release pent-up emotions and embrace your body's changes.
- **Make a powerful playlist:** Create a playlist of songs that make you feel empowered as a woman. These songs should remind you of your strength, resilience, and inner beauty. Play it whenever you need a confidence boost or just want to dance around your living room.

In this chapter, we've explored the myriad of emotions that come with menopause, from the highs to the lows, the laughter to the tears. Remember that it's entirely okay to feel the way you do. Emotions are the vibrant colors that paint the canvas of our lives, and during menopause, that canvas gets a whole lot more interesting!

As we venture into the next chapter, let's recognize that this journey isn't just about personal growth; it's also about the evolution of our connections with others. Just like we're changing, our relationships are, too.

So, get ready to navigate the twists and turns of maintaining, strengthening, and perhaps even redefining your relationships as you embrace your newfound confidence and self-discovery. Let's dive into the depths of how menopause transforms our connections with others and discover new horizons together.

Chapter 4
Hormones and Harmony

Cameron Diaz, mother, actress, and author, was quoted as saying,

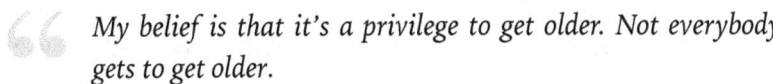 *My belief is that it's a privilege to get older. Not everybody gets to get older.*

Ladies, it's time to get serious about the dynamic of relationships during menopause, because boy, can they get interesting! Here's a woman named Michelle who's been married for years. She hits the big 5-0, and suddenly, her life explodes. She's not alone in this journey. According to Newson Health Research and Education, 7 out of 10 women experiencing marriage difficulties found menopause contributed to their divorce or marriage problems (Hampson, 2022).

Michelle's Story

At the age of 50, she was at a music festival with ten of her closest friends, and she ended up falling into bed with a colleague, whom she affectionately refers to as "Mr. W." She found herself hungover, face down in regret, eventually filing for divorce, and, in her own words, becoming "a crazy person."

Her first-hand experience with menopausal symptoms was nothing short of intense. She couldn't sleep, had mood swings and anxiety that left her crying in bathroom stalls at work or in the mall, and felt like her world was spinning out of control.

But that's not all. In the midst of all this, Michelle was also raising two small girls—one with special needs—and taking care of her 91-year-old mother, who had Alzheimer's and a talent for throwing objects at her head multiple times a day.

Michelle belongs to what she calls "the triple M generation—middle-aged mamas in menopause." They are juggling jobs, parenting, and caregiving for their aging parents. "We've put our careers first, married later, and had children in our 30s, which means we're tackling the challenges of menopause while dealing with teens, tweens, and aging parents. It's like we're trying to juggle chainsaws while making dinner, and we're not even sure how we ended up in the circus."

When Michelle first began feeling "off," she sought help from doctors, lots of them suspecting menopause. But the response she received was disappointingly consistent: "Eliminate alcohol, sugar, and caffeine; go on walks; do yoga; get more sleep; and eat a lot of kale." It was as if the medical community had a checklist, and she was just another box to tick. There was zero education to offer on menopause. Her husband hadn't provided much support either, offering to run a bath in between leaving her to-do lists and rolling his eyes when she was too tired for sex.

She tried to lean on a few friends. Shockingly, this came with a mixed bag. Her best friend, over a few too many glasses of wine, simply recounted all of the horrible physical symptoms to expect. "Did you know this hellscape can last for 10 years?" she would slur.

Chapter 4

Michelle left her place feeling worse and defeated. Her other friends didn't have any more information than she did. Her world was turning upside down.

Michelle knew she had to do something. After divorcing her husband and making some significant changes in how she interacted with most people in her life—putting up those essential boundaries and surrounding herself with those who could offer positivity and support—she saw a shift.

And that's where we come in with this chapter. It's time to discuss how you will change during menopause and what to expect from your relationship dynamics. You won't be the same wife, mother, or friend—and guess what? That's perfectly okay! No, this doesn't mean you can expect drastic measures like divorce or abandoning lifelong friendships. What it means is that you will learn to acknowledge what you need. This chapter will guide you on how to be flexible and communicate effectively as you navigate these sometimes choppy waters.

So, if you've ever felt isolated and misunderstood by your friends and family while going through menopause, fear not. This chapter is here to help you grow together, adapt, and thrive during this incredible journey of change. Let's dive in and have some laughs along the way!

Full-Circle Framework Component #3: Social Dynamics

We're diving headfirst into the world of relationships during menopause! We're going to dissect all the oh-so-relatable changes that happen during this time. We'll talk about those intimate ups and downs in the bedroom—spoiler alert: it's like trying to navigate the desert in the dark. And, as if that's not enough, we'll also look at how your self-image and confidence do a little tango of their own, affecting how you show up for your partner and everyone else. So, grab your sense of humor because we're about to embark on a no-holds-barred exploration of how menopause can turn your social life into a dramedy.

Changes With Partners

So, you're going through menopause, and guess what? Your partner is going through it, too, just in a different way. Let's talk about some of the common changes that might crop up in your relationship:

Emotional Changes

First off, mood swings, irritability, and anxiety are like the triple threat of menopause. Your hormones are playing a game of roulette, and sometimes it feels like they're conspiring against you. One minute, you're the calm and collected queen of serenity, and the next, you're ready to unleash a fiery dragon on anyone who dares to cross your path. Your partner might need a crash course in mood decoding just to keep up!

But, hey, we're all humans, right? You might find it a tad tricky to communicate effectively when you don't understand what is happening either. You may feel more sensitive or less patient than usual, which can lead to misunderstandings or full-on battles over who left the toilet paper roll empty.

Advice: Don't leave them in the dark. Even if you don't have all of the answers, let them in on what you are experiencing. "I am sorry, I am all over the map. I can't explain any of it yet. It may be helpful if you do your own research on menopause. It could help you understand why all of this is happening."

Chapter 4

Sexual Changes

Now, let's get to the juicy stuff. Menopause can be like a foghorn sounding off in the bedroom. Changes in libido, vaginal dryness, and discomfort during intercourse might make you feel like you're starring in your very own dry comedy show. But fear not, my friends! It's not the end of your sex life; it's just a new chapter.

Far too often, we are conditioned to believe that menopause signals the end of our sex lives. I do understand that in those moments of being soaked in your own sweat or sobbing over an empty milk carton, sex is the last thing on your mind. This, too, shall pass. Yes, sex is changing. As we continue through this journey, we just need to shake things up. Think of it as a challenge to get creative and rediscover what makes your engines rev. Lubricants and open conversations with your partner will be your best friends. And who knows? Maybe this phase will unleash your inner sex goddess, and you'll find yourself trying things you never thought you would. The key is to keep the lines of communication open and maintain a sense of humor in the boudoir. After all, laughter is a fantastic aphrodisiac.

Remember that your partner is also getting old. There, I said it. We often get in our heads that we are aging and our sex drive is changing, yet our partners are not. Keep reminding yourself to talk to them. I don't doubt that they, too, are struggling with their own issues. Maybe they are worried about what you are thinking about them under the sheets. Crack open a bottle of wine or order your favorite pizza and have a good chat. You know each other best, and knowing what to expect and how to embrace it will keep you both feeling close.

Self-Image Changes

Menopause can make you question everything, from your changing body to your newfound appreciation for stretchy pants. Your self-image might do a little dance during this time, and that's perfectly normal.

But remember, confidence is still your middle name. Don't let menopause steal your swagger! Embrace the changes and show off your growing wisdom with pride. Your partner fell in love with you for a reason, and that reason isn't going anywhere.

Not a single one of us leaves this world as we entered it. At 80, you and your partner will not be the same people you were when you first met. This just isn't realistic. Have those great conversations and laughs about aging. Make it normal; make it relatable. Remember, it is society that has given us those ridiculous expectations. You will both feel more relaxed knowing you can enjoy this time in your life by just focusing on the great things instead of you sucking in that meno-belly or him stressing about his bald spot.

So, ladies, there you have it: the not-so-glamorous side of menopause in relationships. It's full of peaks and valleys, but with humor, open communication, and a sense of adventure, you can keep the flame burning and continue to enjoy the journey together. Menopause isn't the end; it's just another chapter in your epic love story. Embrace it, laugh through it, and keep sizzling—because you're hotter than ever!

Changes With Friends

Let's say you and your squad have been inseparable for years. You've laughed together, cried together, and even danced your hearts out together at questionable 80s-themed parties. But now, as you hit the menopausal milestone, it's like someone threw a curveball into your friendship dynamic. Don't panic; this is simply part of the thrilling adventure called life.

As we venture through this menopausal maze, our interests and priorities can take a U-turn faster than you can say "hot flash."

Chapter 4

Suddenly, you might find yourself swapping out your Friday night wine-tasting for a cozy evening with a good book or a yoga class that leaves you feeling as flexible as a pretzel. And guess what? That's totally okay!

As your interests evolve, you might notice that you're not as keen on the same activities as your friends anymore. It's like discovering a new flavor of ice cream—you didn't see it coming, but now you're obsessed with it.

You have to be okay with drifting away from those nights of clubbing and starting to seek out friends who share your newfound passions. Maybe you seek things that fuel your soul, like pottery. Have you bonded with a couple of women at a class recently? Now that you've had more free time, maybe you've started exploring your passion for photography. Perhaps you joined a group that meets up once a week. As your needs and wants change, so may your friendship group.

For example, in my 20s, I loved going to see live bands. It didn't matter if they were local or not; I would jump in the car with friends and fall back into bed at 3 a.m. Just thinking about this now exhausts me. I've become sound-sensitive. If I am going to be up past 11, I need a week to prepare. No joke. This doesn't bother me; I just find joy in new things now. Some of the friends I enjoyed live music with stayed there and still love that scene. I am okay with that.

You won't say goodbye to all of those lifelong friends. There will be some you lean on for support during menopause. Menopause might have you reaching out for that comforting chat where you can spill your guts without fear of judgment. You will have those friends who will become your confidantes, cheerleaders, and therapists, all rolled into one fabulous package.

While you're navigating the wild waters of menopause, don't forget to be there for your friends, too. They might be going through their own life changes, whether it's career shifts, relationship bumps, or even their own menopausal adventures. So, keep the wine—or herbal tea—nights on the calendar, even if they're a little less wild than before.

In the end, remember that many friendships do get better with age. Embrace the changes in your relationships with open minds and a heart full of love. Menopause is just another chapter in the book of life, and your friends are right there with you, turning the pages and laughing through every twist and turn. Cheers to friendship and menopausal madness!

Changes With Family

I would like to explore the topic of how your relationship with your family, especially your children, is going to change during menopause. Spoiler alert: It's not all doom and gloom, and there's a lot of room for laughter and growth.

As children grow up and become more independent, you might find yourself in a completely different role as a mother. Gone are the days of endless soccer practices, diaper changes, and helping with homework. Now, your kids are off to college, starting their careers, or maybe even starting families of their own. And guess what? This shift can bring up a whole lot of emotions.

You might experience something commonly referred to as "empty nest syndrome." It sounds like a sad, dusty old bird's nest, right? This one hit me hard. After giving all of myself to raising my children, once they left, I no longer knew what my role was.

I would like you, instead, to think of it as an empty canvas. It's a time of transition, and yes, it can be challenging. I chose to think of it as time for me. I could refocus my time and energy on what fueled my soul.

You may feel a sense of loss, emptiness, or even loneliness as your kids spread their wings and leave your cozy mom cave. But remember, it's not the end; it's a new chapter.

Now, here's the cool part: Menopause can be an opportunity to redefine yourself in your relationships, especially with your children. This is your time to shine, explore your passions, and discover what makes you tick. You've spent years focusing on your kids, your spouse, and your career—now it's time to focus on *you*.

Menopause doesn't mean you're becoming irrelevant or fading into the background. In fact, it's an opportunity to step into the spotlight. Embrace your age, wisdom, and newfound freedom. Be the fabulous, confident, and empowered woman you were always meant to be.

As your kids grow, they'll also see you in a new light. They'll witness your journey through menopause and the way you handle it with grace, humor, and resilience. Trust me; they'll admire and respect you even more for it. Your relationship with them will evolve into something beautiful and different, but no less meaningful.

I cannot help but think of one of my closest friends. She graduated from college but chose to be a stay-at-home mom to her three beautiful children. After 20 years, she had no clue what to do next. She took a brave step at 51 years old and went back to school. By the age of 55, she had become a psychotherapist. I cheered so loudly at her graduation, and my eyes poured tears of pride for her. You see, at any age, you can choose your path.

So embrace this new chapter with unlimited possibility. Use it as an opportunity to rediscover yourself and reclaim your identity. Your relationship with your family, especially your children, is about to transform in ways you never imagined. And you know what? It's going to be one heck of a ride.

Strengthening Bonds

Strengthening all of these bonds while they are changing is going to be important, but how? Well, first, active listening. Trust me; it will help. When your partner or loved one starts sharing their thoughts or feelings, put down the phone and give them your full attention. This is what you would expect, right?

Next, you want to avoid interrupting and resist the urge to jump in with your own story. Ask follow-up questions to show that you're engaged and interested in what they're saying. It's like a verbal hug, and it can go a long way in making them feel heard and valued.

You will want to follow this up by expressing gratitude. Regularly acknowledge and appreciate the positive aspects of your relationships. Even when there are challenges, make a conscious effort to find the silver lining. Try to see things from their point of view—it fosters empathy and leads to more constructive conversations. Plus, who doesn't love a little gratitude sprinkled into their day? For example, despite the fact that your partner may have ignored all the signs that you haven't had a good night's sleep in a month, thank them for picking up the slack around the house or picking up the groceries.

Now, let's dive into open and honest communication. The journey through menopause is demanding, and your loved ones need to know what's going on with you. As I mentioned earlier, even when you don't have all the answers, be open and honest about how you're feeling and what you're experiencing. Encourage them to do the same. This way, you can prevent misunderstandings and build trust. It is the foundation of a strong relationship. It is also okay to say, "I am a mess right now and just need space. This is no reflection of my feelings for you; I just need to catch my breath."

The unbelievable hormonal changes during menopause present us with mood swings and irritability. They just do; there is no escaping it. It's like PMS decided to make a comeback and bring all of their friends. So, practice patience, not just with others but also with yourself. Remember, it's okay to have those moments. We all do. Acknowledge it for what it is and give yourself sympathy, rest, and anything else you need to ride the wave.

Flexibility and adaptability are your allies. Be willing to adapt and make changes to your relationship dynamics if necessary. Maybe it's time to explore new ways of being intimate with your partner, or perhaps you could find some new activities to enjoy with your friends. Change can be exciting, too!

Lastly, seeking support is a courageous move. If you find that navigating relational changes during menopause is particularly difficult, don't hesitate to reach out to a therapist or join a support group. It's like having a squad of cheerleaders who totally get what you're going through.

So, let's embrace these relationship changes with excitement and the power of positivity. We've got the tools to strengthen our bonds, and we're going to emerge from this chapter of life even more fabulous and connected than before. You're a force to be reckoned with, and menopause is just another adventure on your incredible journey!

Chapter 4 Challenge: Keeping Family and Friends Close

Take some time and look over these relatable tips for maintaining and improving communication during this transformative period. Let's review them:

- **Have regular bonding time:** Think of it as a date with yourself or your loved ones. Make it a ritual to connect, laugh, and enjoy each other's company. It's a fantastic way to keep the connection strong.
- **Don't resent what they don't know:** Remember, your friends and family can't read your mind. If something's bothering you or you need support, don't expect them to magically understand. Speak up!
- **Address your feelings ASAP:** If you're feeling a certain way, don't let it fester. Talk about it sooner rather than later. You're a warrior; confront those feelings head-on!
- **Avoid name-calling, blaming, and comparing:** Let's keep it classy, ladies. A good, old-fashioned argument can turn into a comedy show if you throw in some creative insults. But seriously, try to express yourself without pointing fingers.
- **Set expectations early on:** Whether it's setting boundaries or discussing your needs, clear communication from the get-go can save a lot of misunderstandings.
- **Try not to take criticism personally:** We're all going through changes, and sometimes our loved ones may not express themselves perfectly. Don't let it shake your confidence.
- **Never list everything they're doing "wrong":** Trust us; they already know. Focus on the positives and what you appreciate about them.
- **Have serious talks in person and privately:** No one wants to hear about your vaginal dryness while they're in the middle of a board meeting. Save those heart-to-hearts for a quiet, private setting.
- **Never go to bed angry:** Life's too short for grudges. Resolve conflicts before hitting the hay. Who knows, makeup sex could be on the horizon!

- **Be curious and ask "stupid" questions:** There's no such thing as a stupid question, especially when you're exploring the mysteries of menopause. Ask away, and you might just learn something new and exciting!
- **Maintain focus during disagreements:** Stay on topic and avoid veering into unrelated territories. Trust me, you don't want to end up arguing about whose turn it is to take out the trash when the real issue is anxiety or fatigue from insomnia.
- **Don't make assumptions:** Assuming you know what someone else is thinking or feeling can lead to misunderstandings. Ask them directly instead.
- **Don't interrupt:** Give your loved ones the space to express themselves fully. You'll appreciate it when it's your turn.
- **Share your problems:** Don't bottle up your concerns. Your friends and family are there to support you, but they can't do that effectively if they don't know what's going on.
- **Don't lie by omission. Stop trying to "win" arguments:** Honesty is the best policy, even if it means admitting you're wrong or unsure. And remember, relationships aren't competitions; there's no prize for being the "winner."
- **Touch more:** Physical touch can be incredibly comforting and reassuring. Hug it out, hold hands, and rediscover the power of touch.
- **Accept that your partner is not you:** We're all unique individuals, and understanding and celebrating those differences can lead to a deeper connection.

We've covered a lot in this chapter about managing changing relationships during menopause. It's no secret that this journey can put our connections to the test, but remember, you're not alone in this. We've laughed, empathized, and shared our experiences because we know that navigating menopause can be a lot.

As you continue on this adventure, keep these communication guidelines close to your heart. They'll be your trusty tools for maintaining and improving your relationships, whether it's with your partner, friends, or even yourself. Remember to cherish those regular bonding moments, address your feelings, and avoid resentment. Be open, honest, and curious about each other, and above all, maintain that sense of humor.

Now, as we venture into the next chapter, we're about to dive into a topic we all need to talk more about: rekindling that sexual fire during menopause. It's perfectly normal to have questions, concerns, and even insecurities about this aspect of your life. But fear not! We're here to empower you with knowledge, understanding, and confidence.

So, get ready to embrace your sensual side, rediscover the pleasure of intimacy, and reignite the sparks of desire. In the upcoming chapter, we'll explore what to expect during menopause, how to navigate the changes, and, most importantly, how to empower yourself to feel sexy, desirable, and confident like never before. Get excited, because the best is yet to come!

Chapter 5
From Fizzle to Sizzle

Actress, activist, and theater director Cynthia Nixon once remarked,

 The freedom that comes from no longer being fertile is huge.

That sounds more like Samantha than Miranda. (If you know, you know.)

It's time to talk about a topic that's as hot as high noon in the Sahara: your sexuality during menopause. I promise, this isn't going to be one of those boring medical journals or a lecture from your well-meaning but slightly clueless gynecologist. No, we're diving headfirst into this subject with humor, heart, and a splash of optimism.

Lisa's Story

A fabulous firecracker in her early 50s, Lisa had always been a powerhouse, juggling career, family, and everything in between, but lately, something was missing. It wasn't the hot flashes, the night sweats, or even the mood swings that were getting to her the most. It was the sizzle in her love life, or rather, the lack of it.

At first, she brushed it off, thinking, *Hey, I've got a whole lot on my plate; maybe it's normal to feel this way.* But as the days turned into weeks and weeks into months, Lisa couldn't deny the growing canyon between her and her partner, Sam. The spark that once lit up their bedroom had dimmed, and Lisa's confidence took a nose-dive as she grappled with these unexpected changes in her body.

Instead of opening up to Sam about her feelings, Lisa did what many of us do when faced with such intimacy issues. She clammed up, and a cold silence settled in their relationship. The distance grew, and both she and Sam found themselves yearning for the connection they once shared. They both missed sex but were afraid to even say the words.

One day, Sam decided they needed to talk. He sat Lisa down, and as they sipped on some wine, he gently broached the subject. Lisa, hesitant at first, decided it was time to break the ice. She opened up about her insecurities, frustrations, and fear of losing the intimacy that had defined their relationship for years.

Their conversation was raw, emotional, and yes, even a little awkward. Lisa had to confess that vaginal dryness was here to stay and wonder how they could overcome it. One word: lube! But it was also a turning point. Instead of shying away from their challenges, they chose to face them head-on. Together, they decided to be open and honest. Sam could no longer snicker at her hot flashes, and he promised to be more understanding. Lisa agreed to tell him when she needed space, and he promised he wouldn't take it personally. All of these things helped them maintain intimacy and connection.

Chapter 5

It worked. Not overnight, of course, but gradually, the sizzle started coming back. Their love life was rekindled, and the bedroom was buzzing with excitement once more.

In this chapter, we're going to dive deep into the world of changing wants and needs, insecurities, and the many challenges that menopause can throw our way. But don't worry; we're also going to explore how you can redefine intimacy and rediscover your sexual confidence, all while having a good laugh along the way.

So, grab your partner, and let's dive into this bittersweet yet heartwarming journey of embracing the sizzle amid the menopausal fizzle. You're in for a wild, liberating, and downright sexy ride.

Full-Circle Framework Component #4: Sexual Empowerment

Now, I don't know about you, but I used to think that menopause was the end of the line for our sex lives. I mean, seriously, the hot flashes, mood swings, and sleepless nights alone could make anyone feel less than sexy. I am here to tell you we have all been lied to! Menopause doesn't mean the end of our sensuality—it's a new chapter in our erotic novel!

Let's dissect those wonderful surprises waiting around the corner for us.

Vaginal Dryness

Oh, the joys of vaginal dryness during menopause! It's like our lady bits decided to pack their bags and take a hike without asking for our permission, leaving us feeling like our undercarriage is drought-stricken. One minute, you don't give sexual intercourse a second thought. You're thinking, *Hey, I've got this. No problemo!* But the next moment, it's as if your vajayjay has been replaced with sandpaper, and even the thought of intimacy sends shivers down your spine for all the wrong reasons.

But, hey, fear not, intrepid explorer of menopause, because there's a whole aisle at the pharmacy dedicated to lubes and moisturizers that will swoop in like your fairy godmother and save the day! These products are the magical elixirs that transform you from the Sahara Desert to a lush, tropical paradise. Picture yourself as a love goddess once more, with confidence that your intimate moments will be smooth, sensational, and satisfying.

And speaking of these lubricious treasures, don't be shy about experimenting with different textures and flavors. After all, variety is the spice of life, right? Who said menopause can't be an adventure in the bedroom? It's like walking into a gourmet restaurant where you're the VIP guest, and the menu is a buffet of pleasure waiting for you to indulge in. Whether you prefer the silkiness of a water-based lube, the long-lasting glide of a silicone-based one, or even a tantalizing flavored option, the choice is yours! You're the captain of this ship, and you're navigating the waters of pleasure with style and finesse.

So, let's raise a toast to the pharmacy aisle saviors that make our menopausal adventures in the bedroom smoother, sweeter, and oh-so-satisfying. Cheers to turning those sandpaper moments into silk sheets of delight and to embracing menopause as the thrilling, pleasure-filled journey it can be!

Vaginal Tightness

Thanks to those pesky low estrogen levels, our trusty vaginas can decide to go all Hulk mode on us, tightening up like they're training for some kind of body-building competition. It's like your lady bits are channeling their inner Arnold Schwarzenegger, flexing those muscles at the entrance and saying, "No entry without a fight!"

What if you're in the middle of the old bedroom tango and your vagina decides to throw a curveball? Suddenly, you're hit with sensations like pain, burning, and soreness, as if you're having a déjà vu moment, thinking they're back in that "first-time" scenario. Um, no thanks! But fear not, because in this menopausal game, lube is our knight in shining armor who swoops in to save the day.

Lube is not simply a necessity; it's a superstar that can transform your intimate moments from uncomfortable to downright enjoyable. Think of it as your VIP backstage pass to pleasure, granting you access to a world of smooth, frictionless sensations. It's like giving your vagina a spa day, complete with soothing massages and relaxation, even when it's in its "bodybuilder" mode.

Menopause may bring its challenges, but it's also an opportunity to discover new ways to make your intimate moments smooth and sensational. And with lube by your side, you're well-equipped to turn your menopausal adventures into a pleasurable journey.

Incontinence

Seriously, who knew that managing your bladder could become such a challenge, right?

But hold on to your superhero capes, because there's absolutely no need to fret. Menopause might bring its quirks, but it also brings stylish solutions that can make you feel like a sexy vixen, ready to tackle any situation with confidence!

Enter super-cute incontinence underwear, the unsung heroes of our menopausal adventures. These little gems are always there to have your back when you need them most. And the best part? They're discreet, comfortable, and, dare I say it, stylish! Say goodbye to those bulky, unflattering pads and hello to sleek and fashionable knickers that make you feel like you're owning the latest runway trend.

Imagine facing those sneezes, belly laughs, and trampoline sessions head-on, knowing you've got your secret stylish backup.

These underoos not only keep you dry and comfortable but also make you feel like a total boss. You're not just tackling incontinence; you're conquering it with style and grace.

So embrace your newfound superpower of staying dry and confident, even in the face of unexpected bladder mishaps. Because in the grand scheme of life, a little incontinence is only a minor inconvenience. You've got this, and you're doing it with style!

Loss of Libido

Ah, the big one—loss of libido or decreased arousal during menopause. It's like our desires packed their bags, went out for groceries, and somehow got lost on the way back home. You find yourself wondering, *Where did my mojo go? Is it hiding in the pantry with the canned goods?*

But here's the exciting part: Menopause is like hitting the reset button for our intimacy. It's like getting a second chance at defining what it means to be intimate, not just with our partners but also with ourselves. Think of it as an opportunity to embark on a thrilling journey of self-discovery, sensuality, and wisdom.

Imagine this moment as a blank canvas waiting for you to paint your desires, passions, and fantasies. It's an opportunity to rediscover what truly turns you on, what sparks that inner fire, and what brings you closer to your partner in ways you never imagined. You're not starting from scratch; you're building on the rich tapestry of experiences and wisdom that life has bestowed upon you.

So, let's embrace this incredible opportunity to explore and experiment, like a scientist in the laboratory of love. Try new things, revisit old favorites, and let your curiosity guide you. Maybe it's trying out new positions, introducing sexy toys into the mix, or even diving into erotic literature to ignite that spark. The possibilities are endless, and you've got all the tools in your sensual toolbox to make them sizzle.

And here's a little secret: Communication is the ultimate aphrodisiac. Open up to your partner about your desires, fears, and fantasies. Let them know that you're on this journey together, and their support and understanding can make the experience even more intimate and thrilling.

Remember, this isn't the end of your passion; it's an opportunity to reinvent it and create a deeper and more meaningful connection with yourself and your partner. So accept your newfound wisdom and sensuality with gratitude. You're not just getting a second chance at passion; you're getting a second chance at embracing your authentic desires and celebrating the incredible woman you've become. Cheers to a sizzling, sensuous, and fulfilling menopausal journey!

These changes don't mean the end of the line for our sexuality or capacity for intimacy. In fact, they can be a springboard to rediscovering what truly excites us. So, here's to reclaiming our confidence, embracing our inner and outer beauty, and laughing in the face of menopause! Menopause is not the end; it's a new beginning. Let's embrace it with all the youthful vitality, confidence, and fabulousness we've got! Cheers to being desirable, lubricated, sexy, confident, and excited about life's endless possibilities!

Redefining Intimacy

First up, have open and honest communication with your partner. We've talked about it before, but let's emphasize it again. Menopause can do a number on our desires, responses, and, well, pretty much everything below the belt. It's perfectly normal for physical changes to mess with our self-esteem, and it's totally okay for your partner to feel a bit lost, too.

Why is it essential to talk about these changes? Well, the lack of communication can lead to feelings of inadequacy, insecurity, and a drop in self-esteem on our end. On the flip side, our partners might be feeling rejected, unattractive, or even questioning if we still desire them. Yikes, right? But we can tackle these issues head-on, ladies.

When it comes to talking to your partner about sex, here are some pointers:

- **Have short, ongoing conversations:** Menopause can bring daily fluctuations in your mood and desire. Instead of waiting for a big, dramatic talk, make space for little chats. A simple Post-It note on the bathroom mirror saying something like, "Feeling a little all over the map today, just need some space, but remember, I love you!" can set a positive tone for understanding and empathy in your relationship. These small, spontaneous gestures keep the lines of communication open.
- **Be direct about what you're feeling:** Honesty is crucial when it comes to discussing your sexual needs and desires. Let your partner know what's happening "down there" and what you need from them. Remember, your vagina needs a voice, too! Share your physical and emotional changes openly. This vulnerability can foster intimacy and help your partner better understand and support you.
- **Explore what would help you feel more comfortable:** Don't be afraid to express your desires and what makes you feel comfortable in the bedroom. Maybe you need more foreplay, a change in your sexual routine, or even some alone time to connect with your own desires. Communication about your needs is a vital step in reigniting the spark in your sexual relationship.

- **Explore other barriers to desire:** Stress, fatigue, and various life factors can significantly impact your libido during menopause. Be open with your partner about what's going on outside the bedroom. Discussing these external factors can help your partner provide emotional support and create a more conducive environment for intimacy.
- **Make room for other kinds of intimacy:** Remember that sex isn't the only way to connect with your partner. Cuddles, kisses, and simply being close can be incredibly fulfilling and help you maintain a strong emotional bond. Focusing on non-sexual intimacy can reduce pressure and allow you to explore other dimensions of your connection.
- **Loop in an expert:** If you find that the challenges you're facing are particularly tough, consider seeking the help of a therapist or a sex expert who specializes in menopause. They can provide valuable insights, strategies, and exercises tailored to your specific needs. Don't hesitate to involve professionals who can guide you and your partner through this journey.

Incorporating these tips into your conversations about sex during menopause can foster understanding, intimacy, and emotional support between you and your partner. Remember, you're in this together, and open communication is key to maintaining a healthy and fulfilling sexual relationship during this phase of life.

Now, here's the fun part: exploring new ways to connect with your partner. Menopause is the perfect time to get creative and rediscover different forms of intimacy. Think of it as a sexual adventure with your lifelong partner!

Try things like:

- **Sensual massages:** Sensual massages can be a fantastic way to reconnect with your partner and ignite those sparks of passion. Set the mood with some soft lighting, soothing music, and scented candles. Take turns giving each other massages, focusing on areas that feel tense or need special attention. Massages not only help relax your body but also build intimacy and trust, setting the stage for more intimate moments.

- **Exploring fantasies:** Sharing your deepest desires and fantasies with your partner can be a thrilling and liberating experience. Menopause can bring about changes in your desires, so it's an excellent time to open up about what truly excites you. You might be pleasantly surprised at your partner's reaction and willingness to explore these fantasies together. Open communication about desires can lead to a deeper emotional connection and more fulfilling intimacy.

- **Role-play:** Role-playing can add a fun and adventurous element to your sex life. It allows you to step outside your comfort zone and embrace new personas. Don't be shy about getting creative—you can be a naughty nurse, sexy spy, or anything else that tickles your fancy. Role-play encourages playfulness and spontaneity in the bedroom, reigniting the passion that might have waned over time.

- **New sexual activities:** Embracing new sexual activities and experiences can be incredibly rejuvenating for your sex life during menopause. Be open to trying different things in the bedroom, whether it's exploring new positions, incorporating sex toys, or experimenting with sensory play. Variety can reignite the passion and excitement you once had, making your intimate moments feel fresh and exhilarating.

Remember that communication with your partner is key. Discuss your desires, boundaries, and comfort levels when trying new things. Consent and mutual enjoyment should always be the top priorities in your sexual exploration. By actively engaging with these suggestions, you can revitalize your sex life during menopause, creating a fulfilling and satisfying intimate connection with your partner.

This journey is about rediscovering yourself and reclaiming your identity. It's about embracing your age while still feeling sexy, confident, and relevant. So, go ahead and have those conversations with your partner, explore new ways to connect, and keep the passion alive. Menopause is not the end—it's a new chapter in your incredibly sexy life!

How to Feel Like the Sexy Woman You Are!

We need to discuss the tricky topic of body image. Menopause often comes with some unexpected changes, like fluctuating emotions, hair loss, and, yes, shifts in our bodies. But guess what? Those changes don't define us, and they certainly don't take away from our fabulousness.

Sure, we might miss the days when our metabolism worked like a well-oiled machine, but let's not forget that our bodies have carried us through some incredible adventures. They've given birth, climbed mountains, danced at weddings, and laughed until our bellies hurt. Menopause is another chapter in this incredible journey, and it's one we can embrace with open arms and open hearts.

Now, here's the thing about poor body image: It comes with some pretty hidden costs. It can affect your self-esteem, your relationships, and even your overall quality of life. So, it's time to kick those negative thoughts to the curb. How, you ask? Start by focusing on the things you love about your body. Maybe it's the way your laughter lights up a room or the strength you've gained from all those years of taking care of business. Remember, confidence and self-love are incredibly attractive, no matter your age or shape.

But here's a secret weapon that can boost your body image and keep your sexuality sizzling: self-pleasure. Yep, we're talking about solo playtime, ladies! It's not just about physical pleasure—although that's a fantastic perk—but it's also about getting to know your body on a deeper level. Menopause can bring some changes in how we experience pleasure, so exploring your desires can help you understand what makes your body tick now.

Self-pleasure isn't just about maintaining sexual function, though that's a big bonus. It's about reclaiming your sense of control and rediscovering your desires. It's a way to remind yourself that you're still a sensual, passionate being who deserves pleasure and satisfaction. So, don't be shy about exploring your pleasure zones, trying out new things, and finding what works best for you.

Menopause doesn't mean the end of your sexual journey; it's a new beginning! Embrace your body, celebrate your sexuality, and remember that you are vibrant, desirable, and utterly fantastic. Don't let anyone tell you otherwise, because you've got this, and menopause is just another chapter in your amazing story of you.

Chapter 5 Challenge: Affirm Your Goddess Status

Let's dive right into something we all need a little boost in: sexual confidence. Trust me, I get it—the physical changes, mood swings, and the occasional brain fog can make us feel like we're stuck on some bizarre rollercoaster ride. It is time to remember that you are a vibrant, incredible, and sexy woman.

Chapter 5

Here are 20 sassy sexual confidence affirmations to help you embrace your sensuality, feel desirable, and take charge of your newfound wisdom (Davis, 2023):

1. "I am a goddess of sensuality, and menopause is my superpower."
2. "My body may be changing, but my sexiness is ageless."
3. "Confidence is my sexiest accessory, and I wear it proudly."
4. "I am the author of my pleasure, and I'm writing a bestseller."
5. "My desires are valid, and I deserve pleasure and satisfaction."
6. "I radiate irresistible allure, and I attract what I desire."
7. "Menopause is a gateway to my sexual renaissance."
8. "My body is my temple, and I worship its beauty and sensuality."
9. "I embrace my inner vixen with a twinkle in my eyes and a wicked smile."
10. "Age is just a number; my passion knows no limits."
11. "I am the captain of my ship, navigating the seas of pleasure."
12. "Menopause is my chance to rediscover my desires and redefine my sexuality."
13. "I am a magnetic force, drawing in love, pleasure, and adventure."
14. "I am confident in my skin, and it radiates with irresistible allure."
15. "My libido is like fine wine, improving with age."
16. "I am the embodiment of beauty, wisdom, and desire."
17. "I choose pleasure, and I savor every moment of it."
18. "My body is my playground, and I explore it with curiosity and delight."
19. "I am not defined by societal standards; I am defined by my inner fire."

20. "Menopause is not the end; it's a new beginning, and I'm ready to embrace it."

Embrace your sensuality, revel in your desires, and know that you are beautiful, desirable, and utterly fabulous at every age. Let's flaunt this menopause like the goddesses we are!

As we close this chapter on rediscovering our sexual desire during menopause, remember that this is only the beginning of a transformative journey. We've learned that our sensuality is ageless, our desires are valid, and our confidence is our sexiest accessory. Now, it's time to dive deeper into our inner selves, tapping into our spiritual growth and reconnecting with the essence of who we are.

In the next chapter, we'll explore the profound ways menopause can be a catalyst for spiritual awakening. We'll embrace our inner wisdom, find solace in self-reflection, and discover a newfound sense of purpose and inner peace. So, grab your spiritual compass, because we're about to embark on an incredible journey of self-discovery and spiritual reconnection. Get ready to uncover the magic that lies within and embrace the full spectrum of your beautiful, evolving self.

Hey there, fellow midlife adventurers!

Of all the Irish poets and playwrights, Oscar Wilde was one of the best. According to ol' Oscar,

> *The only thing to do with good advice is to pass it on. It is never of any use to oneself.*

Now that we're about halfway through this book, I want to thank you for choosing it and offer a little something to ponder: Have you ever received a recommendation that turned out to be a game-changer for you? Maybe it was a restaurant, a movie, or even a life-

Chapter 5

changing book. Now, think about how awesome it would be if you could be that game-changer for someone else.

Now, I know we're all running around with our hair on fire, but stick with me for a sec because there's something truly special about this book. It's not just about surviving the change; it's about embracing it, using it to rediscover who you are, and reigniting the passions that might have taken a little hiatus.

So here's the thing–I know you're busy conquering the world and all, but you've got a ton of valuable experiences under your belt. Ever think about how your words could be the guiding light for someone else going through a similar journey? Let me drop some truth bombs on you. Your thoughts and experiences matter, and your review could unlock someone else's journey to rediscovery—pretty cool, right? Your insights can be a virtual hand reaching out to someone in need, saying, "Hey, I've been there; you're not alone."

Your words have the power to help someone decide if this book is the missing piece they've been searching for. So, how amazing would it be to know you played a part in someone else's transformative journey?

So, my audacious and daring friend, here's my ask: Could you take a few minutes to leave an honest review of *Fierce and Fab*? And here's a little extra motivation for you: by leaving a review, you're contributing to a community of midlife warriors who uplift and support each other.

Your words matter more than you know.

Cheers to the power of women supporting women!

Chapter 6
Sacred Wisdom in the Second Act

Eliza Farnham was a 19th-century American novelist, feminist, abolitionist, and activist for prison reform. In her lofty rhetoric, she proclaimed:

> *And for her true womanhood arrived here, there is no growing old. Age refines and enriches, warms and illuminates, expands and exalts her. She is more and more Woman through it, not less and less. The noble life that has let her hither is her grand cosmetic. Her intellect, loosed from the golden bonds of corporeal Maternity, rises to the grasp of higher truths.*

Wait, what? Let's break that down into modern English: Once she high-fived her true womanhood, the aging rollercoaster turned into a slapstick joyride. Time threw confetti all over her, making her sparkle and shine like a cartoon character hitting the jackpot. She didn't downgrade her woman status; if anything, she leveled up. Free from the diaper-changing Olympics, her brain did some superhero power-ups, unlocking the mysteries of the universe like a boss.

Ladies, imagine this: a woman, much like you and me, navigating the tumultuous seas of menopause. She's reached a point where she feels adrift, caught in the crossfire of hot flashes and hormonal hurricanes. The chaos in her body is mirrored by the chaos in her mind as she grapples with questions about her purpose, her connection to herself, and the vast, mysterious universe beyond.

One day, in the midst of this whirlwind, our protagonist stumbles upon an opportunity—a chance to attend a spiritual retreat. Now, before you start imagining incense-laden rooms and chanting monks, let's keep it real. This isn't some magical journey where she suddenly levitates into the cosmos or becomes a Zen master overnight. No, my friends, this is about a woman searching for something, anything, to reignite her sense of self and purpose during this transformative phase of life.

As she steps onto the path of the retreat, our brave adventurer is met with a room full of fellow travelers, all in various stages of the menopausal odyssey. Together, they start on a path, not into the mystical realms of unicorns and rainbows, but into the depths of their own souls.

Through meditation, soul-searching conversations, and maybe a few awkward yoga poses, our heroine begins to reconnect with herself on a profound level. She starts to peel back the layers of societal expectations and rediscover the essence of her own being. It's not about becoming someone else; it's about unearthing the hidden gems buried beneath the rubble of daily life.

During one particularly starlit evening, under a sky so vast it makes you question your place in the universe, something miraculous happens. Our woman has had a spiritual awakening. Now, before you roll your eyes and think she's started levitating after all, let me clarify. Her awakening is not about transcending the human experience but embracing it fully. She realizes that she is part of something much greater—a cosmic dance of energy and consciousness that connects us all.

With this newfound awareness, she returns from the retreat, not as a guru on a mountaintop, but as a woman with a sparkle in her eye and a renewed sense of purpose. She incorporates simple spiritual practices into her daily life, like mindful breathing, gratitude journaling, and moments of quiet contemplation. And guess what? She starts to feel like herself again, only better—more confident, more vital, and more in tune with the rhythms of life.

So, my menopausal mavens, as we dive into this chapter on spiritual growth during menopause, remember that it's not about becoming someone else or escaping reality. It's about rediscovering the beautiful, cosmic, and awe-inspiring being you've always been. We're going to explore how you can deepen your connection to yourself and the universe and find that renewed sense of purpose and fulfillment you've been longing for. Get ready to embrace the cosmic connection, because menopause is not the end; it's a cosmic rebirth.

Full-Circle Framework Component #5: Spiritual Connection

It's time to explore the spiritual side of this crazy journey called menopause. Fasten those seat belts, because we're about to embark on a joyful and enlightening ride.

You know, they say menopause is like a popcorn machine in the middle of a romantic movie marathon. Just when you think you've settled into a cozy evening, it starts popping off unexpectedly. You'll laugh, you'll cry, and you'll wonder if it's ever going to stop! But in the end, you'll savor the unique flavor of this cinematic adventure and maybe even find a few surprise kernels of wisdom along the way!

It's also a profound spiritual awakening. Now, I know what you're thinking: *Spirituality? Isn't that for monks on mountaintops or yoga gurus in Bali?* Well, hold on to your leak-proof bloomers, because menopause is here to shake things up, spiritually speaking.

Consider this: You're in the midst of those mood swings, night sweats, and the occasional "I can't find my car keys" moments. But in the middle of all that chaos, something is happening deep within you. It's like a shift in consciousness, a cosmic wake-up call. You start to see the world through different eyes.

Suddenly, you're hit with a deepening of empathy and compassion. You realize that everyone, and I mean everyone, is fighting their own battles. Your heart opens up, and you find yourself extending a helping hand or a kind word to others in a way you never did before.

And that sense of interconnectedness with the universe? Oh, it's real, my friends. You start to notice the beauty in everyday moments. The way the sun sets, the rustle of leaves in the wind, the laughter of children—it all becomes more meaningful. You're in tune with the cycles of life, like the changing seasons, and you realize that you, too, are a part of this grand cosmic dance.

Now, why is it important to embrace this spiritual side of menopause? Well, let me tell you. During this time, you're faced with some deep, soul-searching questions:

- **Reflecting on life's purpose:** You start pondering your life's purpose beyond raising kids or climbing the corporate ladder. Menopause makes you question what truly matters to you.

- **Connecting with inner wisdom:** You tap into a well of wisdom within you that you might not have known existed. It's like finding an ancient treasure chest of insights.
- **Letting go of attachments:** Menopause teaches you to shed the baggage of societal expectations and embrace who you really are.
- **Embracing self-acceptance:** You begin to love and accept yourself unconditionally, flaws and all.
- **Exploring spirituality:** You may find yourself delving into spiritual practices, whether it's meditation, yoga, or simply spending time in nature.
- **Connecting with nature and the cycles of life:** You become attuned to the natural rhythms of the world and see the beauty in its ebb and flow.
- **Reevaluating priorities:** Menopause forces you to reexamine what truly matters in your life. Hint: It's not about the number on your birthday cake.
- **Seeking support and community:** You seek out like-minded women who are on this journey with you, forming a powerful support network.
- **Finding meaning in aging:** You start to realize that aging isn't a curse but a privilege. Each wrinkle and gray hair tells a story of a life well-lived.

"Pregnant women give birth to new souls. Menopausal women give birth to their wiser selves (Sharratt, 2019)." We're not just fading into the background. Menopause is like a cosmic invitation to live in harmony with the tides and seasons of our lives. It's a time to embrace our inner wisdom, share our newfound compassion, and rediscover ourselves in the process.

So, let's raise a glass to the spiritual awakening that menopause brings. It's a difficult climb, but oh, the view from the top is worth it! Embrace the spiritual aspects of this transition and let your wiser self shine.

The Natural Rhythm of Life

Let's talk about menopause and how it parallels the natural seasons of life. But wait, before we get into the nitty-gritty, grab your favorite snack and a drink, because we're about to have a great chat about this rollercoaster ride called menopause.

Menopause is Mother Nature's way of giving us a front-row seat to her spectacular show. You know, just like how the seasons change, so do our bodies. It's like going from summer to fall to winter... and then, spoiler alert, there's a spring waiting for us on the other side!

Now, let's talk about menopause as our personal winter. Yep, winter. It's not the end of the world; it's just a season, ladies. Sure, it might come with its fair share of snowstorms (hot flashes) and slippery sidewalks (mood swings), but it's also a time for introspection and renewal.

Think about it: Winter forces us to slow down, to take stock of our lives. A hush falls over the land. The trees shed their leaves, and a quiet blanket of snow covers the ground. It is a time for quiet, a time for pause. Similarly, menopause allows us to reflect on the journey we've been on so far. It's like our bodies are saying, "Hey, remember those dreams and desires you put on hold while raising kids, climbing the career ladder, or just dealing with life? Well, now's the time to dust them off."

As the world outside becomes quieter, it's a perfect opportunity to listen to your inner voice. What have you always wanted to do but never had the time for? Travel more? Start a new hobby? Learn to tap dance? Write that novel you've been daydreaming about?

Chapter 6

Menopause isn't only about looking inward; it's also about adapting to change. Nature teaches us this lesson, too. Trees let go of their leaves in the fall, birds migrate, and animals hibernate. Life constantly evolves, and so do we. We must learn to embrace the changes and let go of what no longer serves us. We were never meant to stay the same forever.

Letting go can be tough. Maybe you're letting go of your youth, the ability to bear children, or the constant need for validation. But trust me, what awaits on the other side of this season is breathtaking.

Just like spring follows winter, there's a renewal that comes with menopause. It's like Mother Nature saying, "Here's your fresh start!" You're not just growing older; you're growing wiser, more confident, and beautifully radiant from the inside out.

With spring comes newness—fresh blossoms, greener grass, and vibrant leaves. When you emerge from your winter, you should expect newness, too. How you embrace this change is pivotal. Try new things, embrace new moments, and create a beautiful, vibrant you.

What can we learn from all of this? Adaptability. Letting go. Renewal. These are the gifts menopause brings, if we're willing to accept them. Just like the trees bloom again in spring, so can you. Find your passions, explore your desires, and reclaim your identity.

And remember, ladies, you are still desirable, sexy, and relevant. Menopause isn't the end; it's a new beginning. Embrace your inner and outer beauty, be proud of the incredible journey you've been on, and get ready to shine brighter than ever before. Menopause might be your winter, but there's a glorious spring just around the corner. Embrace it with enthusiasm, and let your fabulous self bloom like the most beautiful flower in the garden.

Expanding the Connection to the Universe

Menopause is a spiritual journey waiting to be explored, and we're here to guide you through it with humor and heart.

Embrace the Divine Feminine

Alright, ladies, you've hit menopause, and your body's waving the "No more babies" flag. It's like your biological clock decided to stop ticking, and that's perfectly okay! In fact, it's time to high-five that divine feminine energy within you.

Menopause isn't the end; it's a spiritual initiation. It's your cosmic promotion to wisdom and intuition. You've gathered all this life experience, and now it's time to tap into your inner oracle, your inner goddess. You see, the ancient cultures knew the power of the Divine Feminine, and now it's your turn to embrace it fully.

Now, let's talk about connecting with your inner goddess. Close your eyes, take some deep breaths, and visualize a powerful, radiant, and wise woman within you. She's been there all along, but now it's time to acknowledge her presence. Feel her energy, strength, and wisdom flowing through you.

Embracing Change

Let's start by questioning the notion that change is something to be feared or resisted. In reality, change is a fundamental part of life, and it's often a catalyst for growth, transformation, and new opportunities. Menopause is a natural part of a woman's life, and it's a profound change, but it doesn't have to be a negative one. Think of it as your golden ticket—a ticket to a new chapter filled with exciting possibilities.

Just like those trees shedding their leaves in autumn to prepare for a fresh start in spring, menopause is your season of transformation. It's a time when you shed what no longer serves you, just like those leaves falling gracefully to the ground. Those fears, insecurities, and outdated beliefs? Let them go like the leaves, making way for new growth.

We live in a society that often portrays aging as something to be fought against—a battle to preserve youth at all costs. But it's time to toss those society-imposed ideas out the window! Embracing menopause means rejecting the notion that aging is a negative process. It's about recognizing that every age brings its own unique beauty and wisdom.

Mindful Awareness

Think of mindfulness as your trusty seatbelt on this hormonal rollercoaster. It's there to keep you safe and grounded as you navigate the ups and downs. Mindfulness is about being fully present in the moment, accepting your feelings and sensations without judgment, and staying in tune with your body.

One of the simplest and most effective mindfulness practices you can embrace is deep breathing. When you feel the heat of a hot flash or the surge of a mood swing, take a moment to pause. Inhale deeply through your nose, counting to four, hold for a second, and then exhale slowly through your mouth for a count of six. Repeat this several times. Deep breathing helps calm your nervous system, ease tension, and bring you back to the present moment.

Mindfulness also nurtures emotional intelligence. It helps you become more aware of your emotions, allowing you to explore and understand them deeply. This emotional awareness can lead to healthier ways of processing and expressing your feelings, fostering better relationships with others, and, most importantly, with yourself.

Connecting With Your Body

It's important to recognize that your body is indeed a temple. It's a magnificent vessel that has carried you through life's adventures and challenges. Now, during menopause, it's time to shift your focus from simply existing in your body to truly appreciating and caring for it. Holistic health practices offer an inclusive approach to well-being, considering the physical, emotional, mental, and spiritual aspects of your being. Here are some holistic practices that can be particularly beneficial during menopause:

- **Herbal remedies:** Explore the world of herbal remedies to support your body's natural balance during menopause. Herbs like black cohosh, red clover, and evening primrose oil are known for their potential benefits in managing menopausal symptoms. Consult with a holistic healthcare provider or herbalist for personalized guidance.
- **Acupuncture:** Acupuncture is an ancient Chinese practice that involves inserting thin needles into specific points on the body to promote energy flow and balance. Many women find relief from hot flashes, mood swings, and insomnia through acupuncture sessions.
- **Aromatherapy:** Aromatherapy involves the use of essential oils from plants to enhance physical and emotional well-being. Essential oils like lavender, geranium, and clary sage can be soothing and help alleviate stress, anxiety, and sleep disturbances.
- **Reiki:** Reiki is a Japanese energy healing technique that aims to balance the body's energy and promote relaxation and healing. Reiki sessions can help you release emotional blockages, reduce stress, and enhance your overall sense of well-being.

Chapter 6

Rituals and Ceremonies

Light a candle, do a self-blessing, or invite friends and family for a sacred ceremony to mark this incredible milestone. Start thinking of it as a blessing, a great honor, and a transition instead of this horrible end. Honor the wisdom and strength you've amassed on your life journey so far. It's like throwing a party for your awesome self!

Self-Compassion

Menopause, let's face it, is no cakewalk. It's a period filled with physical changes, emotional ups and downs, and adjustments to a new phase of life. Sometimes, it might feel like you're navigating uncharted waters, and that's perfectly normal.

During these changes and challenges, it's vital to be as kind to yourself as you would be to your best friend. Imagine how you'd comfort and support your closest friend going through a tough time. Now, apply that same compassion and understanding to yourself.

You are not alone in this journey. You have permission and the right to seek support when needed. Whether it's talking to a therapist, seeking advice from a healthcare provider, or confiding in a trusted friend or family member, reaching out for support is a sign of strength, not weakness.

One of the most important things to remember is that there's no need to rush through menopause. This is your unique journey, and it unfolds at its own pace. There's no set timeline, and there's no right or wrong way to experience it. Embrace each moment, whether it's a good day or a miserable day, as a part of your story.

Exploring Inner Wisdom

Menopause is often referred to as the "change of life," and for good reason. It's a significant transition that signals the end of one phase and the beginning of another. During this time, your body, mind, and spirit are undergoing profound changes, which can naturally lead to introspection and self-reflection.

One of the most effective tools for introspection is journaling. Grab a notebook or create a digital journal and let your thoughts flow freely onto the pages. Write about your experiences, emotions, hopes, and fears. Journaling allows you to explore your thoughts and feelings in a safe and private space, making it easier to gain insights into your journey.

As you engage in these introspective practices, you'll begin to tap into your inner wisdom and intuition. Your inner wisdom is the accumulation of your life experiences, lessons learned, and innate knowledge. Your intuition is the deep, gut-level feeling that guides you in making choices aligned with your true self. Menopause provides a unique opportunity to reconnect with these sources of inner guidance.

Healing From Within

Emotional baggage from the past may pop up during menopause. It's an opportunity to heal and let go. Consider talking to a therapist or exploring energy healing practices like Reiki. It's like a spa day for your soul!

Embracing New Passions

As you sail into this new phase of life, let your passions run wild. Whether it's painting, traveling, volunteering, or learning something new, follow your heart. Your newfound interests are like sparks of stardust lighting up your life.

Chapter 6

Building a Supportive Community

Surround yourself with kindred spirits who get you. Join women's circles, spiritual groups, or online communities where you can share, learn, and inspire others. Together, you'll conquer the cosmos of menopause.

Menopause is more than a biological event; it's a cosmic awakening! It's a journey of self-discovery, healing, and empowerment. As you navigate this cosmic rollercoaster, remember to cherish your body, nurture your mind, and connect with your spirit. Seek guidance and support from your spiritual community and holistic practices. You'll find that menopause is a profound, spiritual, and fulfilling adventure.

And don't forget about nature—it's your ultimate cosmic classroom. Spend time in its embrace, observe its rhythms, and gain insights into your menopausal voyage. Take a leisurely nature walk, meditate under a tree, get your hands dirty, practice yoga in the great outdoors, or even start a garden. Nature's wisdom is like the universe's best-kept secret, waiting for you to uncover it.

The universe is calling. Embrace the journey, shine like the star you are, and remember, age is just a number—your cosmic number!

Chapter 6 Challenge: The Menopause Release Ritual

We're about to embark on a journey that's going to empower you through a little something I like to call the Menopause Release Ritual. Now, I know what you're thinking, *A ceremony for menopause? Really?* But trust me, it's not your grandma's ritual. This is all about embracing the change and letting go of the baggage that comes with it. So, let's dive right in!

Before we get started, let's talk about what a menopause ceremony is. It's not some stuffy, formal event with robes and incense—unless you're into that, in which case, go for it! It's more like a personal, symbolic celebration of your transition into this exciting phase of life. It's a way to mark the occasion and release all those pesky fears, insecurities, and old beliefs that have been holding you back.

You might be wondering why this is even important. Well, my fabulous friends, it's important because it's all about reclaiming your power and embracing your new self. Menopause is not the end; it's a new beginning! This ritual will help you let go of those nagging doubts and make space for fresh, positive vibes and intentions.

Instructions for Your Release Ritual

Preparation

Find a quiet and comfy space where you won't be disturbed. Think cozy blankets, a cup of herbal tea, and maybe even some soothing music. Grab some paper and a pen, and if you're feeling adventurous, a small fire-proof container—a metal bowl or even a heat-resistant dish—will do. Oh, and before you start, take a few deep breaths to center yourself. You're about to embark on something transformative!

Reflection

Now, close your eyes and reflect on those fears, insecurities, and old beliefs that have been buzzing around in your head like pesky mosquitoes. Is it the fear of aging? Insecurities about your changing body? Maybe those old beliefs about what menopause means for you? Take your time with this. Be gentle with yourself. You're in no rush.

Chapter 6

Writing

Next, grab that pen and write down everything you wish to release. And I mean everything! Be specific, my friend. Write each fear, insecurity, or belief on separate pieces of paper. There's something liberating about seeing those thoughts on paper.

Release

Now comes the fun part! Safely burn those pieces of paper in your fire-proof container or, if you prefer, tear them up and toss them away. As you do this, visualize those fears, insecurities, and beliefs being transformed and released into the universe. Watch them disappear like smoke in the wind.

Affirmation

After you've let go of it all, stand tall and say a positive affirmation out loud. Something like, "I release the past and welcome the new, positive energies into my life." Say it with conviction, like you mean it, because you do!

And there you have it—your very own menopause release ritual. It's a moment to celebrate your journey, embrace your newfound confidence, and let go of anything that's been holding you back. You are desirable, sexy, confident, and relevant, my dear. This ritual is just one step on the path to rediscovering yourself and reclaiming your identity. So, go forth, fabulous woman, and let the world see your inner and outer beauty shine!

In this chapter, we've embarked on the wild and wacky ride called menopause, and guess what? It's a time of profound spiritual growth. Who knew? Menopause isn't Mother Nature's way of playing a hormonal prank on us; it's a cosmic invitation to discover our inner Zen master.

Fierce and Fabulous After Menopause

We've dabbled in practices like meditation, which, let's face it, sometimes feels more like trying to herd cats than achieving inner peace. And don't get me started on journaling—scribbling down your thoughts might seem like deciphering ancient hieroglyphs at times. But you know what? Amid the chaos, menopause offers us a golden ticket to connect with our inner wisdom and intuition.

Yes, ladies, it's time to rekindle the flames of our inner goddess. Who knew she was lurking there, just waiting for menopause to nudge her awake? With a newfound spiritual awareness that's as surprising as finding your car keys in the freezer, we're ready to tackle the next chapter of our journey: freedom!

Menopause might have thrown us for a loop, but it's not a life sentence. It's more like a get-out-of-jail-free card from the Monopoly game of societal expectations and limitations. Let's flip the page and dive into the liberating sense of freedom that's waiting for us in the chapters ahead. Get ready to spread those wings, ladies, and soar into the post-menopausal world like the fabulous phoenixes we are. Life's too short to let menopause steal our sparkle, so let's shine on!

Chapter 7
From Restrained to Radiant

Let's hear what American author Akiko Busch has to say and what most women over 50 have experienced:

 As they age, women experience less public scrutiny–and entertain a wider set of choices about when and how they are seen.

You know that moment when you're standing in your empty nest, waving goodbye to your kids as they head off to college? Yeah, it's a bittersweet mix of pride and sadness. But it's also the moment when menopause decides to waltz into your life unannounced. Just when you thought you had enough on your plate with the kids gone, your hormones decide it's time to throw a wild party of their own.

So, there I was, feeling like my life was suddenly adrift. The house that once echoed with the morning chaos of kids getting ready for school now felt eerily quiet. And on top of that, my body seemed to be staging a mutiny. Sleepless nights, anxiety, and added weight gain were now my new, unwanted roommates.

What I have learned is that menopause, as it turns out, isn't just about losing things—it's also about finding yourself in the process. With the house quieter than ever, I decided it was time to make some noise of my own. I signed up for that pottery class I had always dreamed of—the one I had put on the back burner for years because of PTA meetings and soccer practices.

As I nervously walked into that first class, I had no idea how it would change my life. But there's something about getting your hands dirty and shaping clay into something beautiful that mirrors the process of rediscovering yourself. I met a bunch of amazing women there, all at different stages of life, but all in search of something more.

Through that class, I found a tribe of kindred spirits who laughed at my menopause-induced anecdotes, shared their own stories, and reminded me that I wasn't alone in this journey. We didn't just mold clay; we formed a bond.

And you know what? The newfound freedom that comes with menopause is a breath of fresh air. It's an opportunity to reinvent, to rediscover, and to reconnect with the parts of yourself that may have been overshadowed by years of nurturing others. It's a time to embrace your inner artist, your inner adventurer, your inner you.

In this chapter, we'll dive into the incredible journey of self-discovery that menopause can be. We'll explore strategies for reinvention, share stories of women who've redefined their lives, and provide you with the tools to find your own passion and purpose. So, get ready to shed the old and step into the new with the confidence and vitality that only come with experience. Your freedom awaits, and trust me, it's a journey worth taking.

Chapter 7

Full-Circle Framework Component #6: Freedom and Reinvention

Who would have thought that the absence of those monthly visitors could bring such joy and liberation? It's like winning the lottery, but without the hassle of taxes or paparazzi.

So, there you are, officially entering the land of menopause, and you suddenly realize that you're no longer a slave to your menstrual cycle. No more stocking up on tampons or wondering if your white jeans are safe to wear. Your uterus is like, "Bye-bye, monthly maintenance," and you're free to kick up your heels in those sassy pants with reckless abandon.

This newfound freedom isn't only about periods; it's about you, glorious you. You start feeling a surge of self-confidence because you've weathered the storm of hormones, mood swings, and cramps for decades. You're basically a superhero without a cape (because capes are so last season).

Empowerment becomes your middle name as you realize that biology no longer defines your worth based on your reproductive potential. You're not a vessel for future generations; you're a full-fledged, amazing person with dreams, goals, and desires. Now is the time to explore them without the pesky hormonal rollercoaster getting in the way.

Oh, and let's not forget about the sweet release of vanity. No more squeezing into biting spanx or fretting about your crow's feet. You've earned every line and wrinkle, and you wear them like badges of honor. Who cares if hair grows in places it shouldn't? You're too busy enjoying the grand scheme of life, my friend.

As you journey through menopause, you might notice a sense of relief as anxiety about unmet ambitions starts to dissipate. That restlessness you once felt? It's like a distant memory, replaced by a newfound sense of calm and contentment. You've got a "been there, done that" attitude, and it's incredibly liberating.

Research shows that people get happier as they get older (Blanchflower et al., 2023). Yep, despite the redistribution of body fat and the occasional groan when you stand up from a low chair. Happiness levels soar, like a phoenix rising from the ashes, as you embrace the incredible freedom that comes with age and experience.

Let's celebrate this glorious phase of life with open arms, bat wings and all. Menopause isn't the end; it's a new beginning, an opportunity to rediscover yourself and reclaim your identity. It's about saying no to the nonsense, embracing your inner and outer beauty, and living life to the fullest. And yes, you can do it all while wearing comfy pajamas or a flowing skirt because comfort and confidence go hand in hand.

Don't be surprised if someone tries to rain on your menopausal parade; haters gonna hate. But for now, let's relish in the joys and the relief. Menopause, you're not so bad after all—you're like the VIP pass to the best party in town!

Reinvention and Rediscovery

As women on that bridge to menopause or deep in the thick of it, we are no strangers to hearing the negatives. I, for one, would like to hear more about reinvention and rediscovery during this exciting phase of life.

Now, we all know that society, family, and tradition have a knack for laying out these neat little paths for us, right? There are these milestones we're supposed to achieve at certain ages and roles we're expected to fill, like clockwork. Menopause gives us a golden opportunity to hit the pause button and ask ourselves some vital questions.

Ask yourself if you have been living a life that's true to your hopes, dreams, and desires. Or, have you just been rolling along on autopilot, following a path you sort of fell into because it seemed like the thing to do? Trust me, this is far too common. You can wake up after 25 years, three kids, a marriage, and wonder how you got there. Menopause is like a wake-up call, my friends. It's time to take stock of your life and make a conscious decision to live it in alignment with your values and passions.

Think of it as unearthing those dreams and desires that might have been gathering dust while you were busy tending to other responsibilities. You know, those passions that were shelved as you raised kids, nurtured a career, or played the role of the dutiful spouse. Now is your opportunity to dust off those dreams and bring them back to life.

But hold on, ladies; we're not here to dwell on the past with regret. Oh, no! Menopause is all about embracing the future with optimism. It's a time of transition, and transitions offer a unique vantage point to see life from a different perspective. So, let's talk about what it means to reinvent and rediscover yourself.

Remember, you've got time on your side. Seriously! You have the gift of experience to guide you. You're not starting from scratch; you're building on a foundation of wisdom and life lessons. Consider yourself a seasoned pro at this reinvention game.

Remind yourself that it's okay to become a student all over again. Dive into your passions with the enthusiasm of a newbie. Learn, explore, and don't be afraid to make mistakes along the way. It's all part of the journey, and you're never too old to learn something new.

Now, don't forget about your support squad—friends and family. They can be your biggest cheerleaders and sources of inspiration. Share your dreams and aspirations with them, and who knows, you might discover that they have some hidden talents and dreams of their own.

I know this entire menopausal journey can leave you feeling like you are floating alone in the middle of the ocean. You need to remind yourself that there's a whole community of women going through the same reinvention process. Connect with them, swap stories, and learn from each other's experiences. It's amazing how empowering it can be to share this journey with others who understand what you're going through.

And don't neglect your past, either. Your life experiences, even the hardest ones, have shaped you into the incredible person you are today. Embrace your history, learn from it, and use it as a stepping stone for your future adventures.

Lastly, understand that reinvention is an ongoing process. It never stops! As you discover new passions, set fresh goals, and achieve amazing things, you'll find that life is a continuous journey of growth and transformation. Don't be afraid to use every tool at your disposal to make those opportunities happen.

Menopause is not the end; it's a thrilling new beginning. It's your opportunity to redefine yourself, reignite your passions, and live a life that's truly your own. So, go ahead, ladies, and reinvent yourselves with gusto.

How to Reinvent and Rediscover Yourself

You've reached this magical stage in life, and it's time to take a step back and evaluate where you're at. I mean, seriously, when was the last time you paused to think about yourself and what makes you tick? Probably somewhere between the first diaper change and your kid's last college tuition payment. Yes, we all know it goes that fast!

But now's the time to dig deep and become aware of what you want and why you don't have it yet. Maybe you've been so busy being a mom, partner, and career rock star that you forgot what your dreams even look like. Let's have a look at some ideas to get you started:

- **Chart a new path:** Let's chart a new path, shall we? Rediscover those long-forgotten passions and dreams. Always wanted to take up painting? Well, grab some brushes and let your inner artist shine! And remember, it's not about being the next Vincent van Gogh; it's about enjoying the process and unleashing your creative side.
- **Identify your life's purposes:** Now, let's dive a bit deeper. What's your life's purpose? I know, I know, it's a big question. But guess what? You have the time and wisdom now to figure it out. Whether it's volunteering, starting a new career, or simply being the best version of yourself, it's time to embrace what truly matters to you.
- **Embrace change and uncertainty:** Menopause is like Mother Nature's curveball, right? Well, don't just dodge it; catch that curveball and run with it. Life is unpredictable, and the sooner we make peace with that, the better. Embrace change and uncertainty in your personal life, and remember, you've got this!
- **Pursue new hobbies or interests:** Let's talk hobbies. Starting a new hobby is like planting a seed of joy in your life garden. Revisit an old one that used to light you up, or try something totally new. Skydiving, surfing, salsa dancing —the choices are endless. And who cares if you're a beginner? The fun is in the adventure!

- **Do something scary:** Speaking of adventures, why not do something a little daring? Go on a trip by yourself or drag a friend along. It's exhilarating to explore new places and cultures, and it's a reminder that you're still that adventurous spirit you were in your youth.
- **Reinvent yourself professionally:** Let's switch gears to your professional life. Maybe you've been on a career hiatus, focusing on other aspects of your life. Well, consider going back to work or starting a business. You've got experience, wisdom, and a fresh perspective to offer—the workforce needs you!
- **Deal with health issues head-on:** Health issues can be a bit of a downer, but don't let them hold you back. Address them head-on and prioritize your well-being. Whether it's a new fitness routine or healthy eating plan or finding ways to manage menopausal symptoms, put yourself first.
- **Elevate your self-care game:** Now, let's give your self-care routine a makeover. It's time to boost that confidence level, ladies! Upgrade your skincare routine with products designed to nourish and rejuvenate mature skin, providing the care it deserves during this significant life stage. Treat yourself to a luxurious facial mask, indulge in a soothing bath, and embrace the natural beauty that comes with embracing the changes in your body.
- **Change your mindset about what you can wear:** First, change your mindset about what you can and cannot wear. Who says you can't wear the hell out of that leather jacket or those skinny jeans? Wear whatever makes you feel confident and fabulous.
- **Experiment with fashion:** Try new colors and styles that you've never worn before. Remember, fashion is all about expressing yourself. Play with it, have fun, shake your tail feathers, and don't be afraid to stand out.

- **Get a new haircut and add some makeup:** Speaking of standing out, a new haircut and a touch of makeup can work wonders for your self-esteem. A fresh look can make you feel like a million bucks, even on the toughest menopausal days.
- **Cut out toxic relationships:** Let's talk about relationships. If you've got some toxic ones hanging around, it's time to Marie Kondo your life and say goodbye to those who don't spark joy. Surround yourself with people who uplift and support you—you deserve it!
- **Cultivate new friendships and reconnect:** Last but not least, cultivate new friendships and reconnect with old ones. It's never too late to build meaningful connections with people who understand your journey. Friends are the secret spice of life, and you deserve a flavorful social circle.

Reinvention and rediscovery are all about embracing your power, celebrating your uniqueness, and living life to the fullest. Menopause may bring challenges, but it also brings opportunities for growth, self-love, and a whole lot of joy along the way.

Women Achieving Greatness After 50

Let's take a closer look at some inspiring stories of women who defied age stereotypes, pursued their passions, and embarked on exciting adventures later in life. These women will remind you that life after menopause can be a thrilling journey full of new achievements and experiences.

Laura Ingalls Wilder

You probably know her as the author of the beloved *Little House on the Prairie* series. But did you know that she didn't start her writing career until her 40s? Laura found publishing success later in life, and her first book, *Little House in the Big Woods*, was published when she was a sprightly 65 (Fields, 2021). Talk about a late bloomer. Her journey to becoming a renowned author wasn't without its challenges, but she never gave up, and her stories continue to captivate generations.

Julia Child

The iconic chef we all adore didn't start her culinary journey until her 30s. It wasn't until she was 50 that she had her own TV show (Seaman, 2022). Julia wasn't afraid to roll up her sleeves, try new things, and live life to the fullest. She embraced joy, adventure, and sensuality (think butter), proving that age is just a number when it comes to pursuing your passions.

Nola Ochs

Talk about lifelong learning! Nola received a Guinness World Record for being the oldest person to earn a college degree, and she did it in 2007 at the impressive age of 95. She took a full course load, lived in student housing, and was a tech-savvy student who operated her computer with ease. Her chosen field of study? History (Green, 2016)! Nola's story reminds us that it's never too late to expand our horizons and chase our educational dreams.

Tamae Watanabe

Climbing Mount Everest is no small feat, and Tamae accomplished it in 2002 at the age of 73, becoming the oldest woman to do so (*Tamae Watanabe, 73, Smashes Own Record as Oldest Woman to Climb Mount Everest*, 2012). Her determination and resilience are awe-inspiring, showing us that age should never limit our pursuit of adventure and conquering new heights—quite literally!

These remarkable women prove that life doesn't end with menopause; it's the beginning of a new and exciting chapter. They embraced change, followed their passions, and proved that you can achieve amazing things at any age. So, my menopausal friends, let these stories inspire you to live your best life, seize every moment, and rediscover the vibrant, confident, and adventurous you that's still very much alive within!

Chapter 7 Challenge: Your Bucket List

I have to admit, I love lists. They help me feel in control and on task. If I am being completely honest, I have been a list maker as far back as I can remember. I get excited at the thought of sitting down and making a grocery list. So, yes, I have made more than one bucket list in my life. I encourage you to do the same!

1. Find a cozy spot where you can relax and reflect. You know, a place where you can let your hair down and truly be yourself.
2. Take a few deep breaths and clear your mind. You might want to put on some soothing music or light a scented candle for ambiance. It's all about setting the mood, my friend.
3. Close your eyes and let your thoughts wander. Reflect on your desires, dreams, and long-term goals. Think about all aspects of your life, from personal development to career, hobbies, and adventure. Nothing is off-limits here.
4. Get a pen and piece of paper, or use your phone, tablet, or computer if you prefer digital. Now, start jotting down all the things you've always wanted to do. Seriously, go wild! Whether it's learning to tango, traveling to a far-off land, writing a book, or simply mastering the art of making the perfect margarita, write it all down.
5. Take a moment to reflect on each item on your list. Do you notice any common themes? Maybe you've got a burning

desire for adventure, a thirst for creativity, or a longing for personal growth. Are there any items that make your heart skip a beat with excitement?

6. Once your list is complete, take a step back and admire it. This is a collection of your dreams and aspirations—the essence of who you are and what you want to experience in this wonderful phase of life. How cool is that?

7. Keep your bucket list somewhere visible—on the fridge, your bedside table, or even as your phone's wallpaper. Let it serve as a daily reminder that life is brimming with possibilities. You are in the driver's seat, and you've got the power to make these dreams a reality.

Remember, this bucket list isn't simply a list; it's your passport to rediscovering yourself and embracing all that life has to offer. It's your way of saying, "I'm here, I'm fabulous, and I'm ready to take on the world!"

As we come to the end of our exciting journey through menopause, it's clear that this phase of life isn't a final curtain call; it's an exhilarating new act in the play of our lives. We've talked about hot flashes, mood swings, and even rediscovering our inner vixen—yes, she's still in there, but we've saved one grand finale act for you, my fabulous menopausal friend: legacy!

Now, I know what you're thinking: *Legacy? Isn't that something for ancient philosophers or famous folks like Shakespeare or Cleopatra?* Well, you're absolutely right, but here's the twist—legacy isn't reserved for history books or pyramid builders. It's for us, too!

As we navigate the sea of menopause, we've unlocked newfound freedom, a zest for life, and a bucket list that's filled with excitement and possibilities.

In the next chapter, we'll look at how you can craft a legacy that perfectly reflects your quirks, passions, and fabulousness. From

Chapter 7

writing a heartfelt letter to your future self—who may be sipping piña coladas on a beach somewhere—to sharing your wisdom with the world—because, let's face it, you've got plenty of it—we'll explore all the fun and meaningful ways to leave your mark.

Chapter 8
Be a Living Legend of Wisdom and Wonder

World-renowned and much-loved Maya Angelou was an American memoirist, poet, and civil rights activist. Getting right to the heart of it, she said:

 If you're going to live, leave a legacy. Make a mark on the world that can't be erased.

Welcome to the last chapter of this life-changing book. You have sweat and plucked your way through with confidence and savvy! I am proud of you. I am on this menopause train with you, so I know staying focused isn't one of our strong suits, but this topic is important. Gaining the knowledge and empowerment we deserve during this time in our lives needs to be more important. So, yes, I am proud of you for making *you* a priority. Job well done!

Tracy's Story

It is the morning after Tracy's family decided to throw her a surprise 50th birthday party. She is awake before everyone else, enjoying a quiet cup of coffee on the porch. Her thoughts are all focused on the same thing. *I am 50. Where in the hell did all the time go?* As she sits there in silence, wrapped in the coziest of blankets, she starts to replay her life.

Married shortly after college—like so many of us did back then—she started her family young. Soon, she would find herself changing diapers, wiping noses, and helping with fifth-grade science projects. That marketing degree she got? It would stay hung on the wall, the frame collecting dust.

She loved being a mother and a wife. She never had that mom who baked cookies and went on school trips. She often walked home to an empty house and snacked on stale chips into the night. She had parents with high-power careers that always seemed to come first. She just wanted to be a different, more available mother.

Yet, now, she sits on her porch—alone. Yes, she was still a mother, but they all left home to begin lives of their own. Yes, she had a partner whom she adored, but she felt empty, like nothing was hers. She couldn't help but think that when she left this earth, how would she be remembered?

Leaving a legacy that her family would talk about for generations was something she was passionate about. Her body may have turned 50 yesterday, but her brain felt 30 and hungry for life. She had spent years volunteering at an animal shelter, always drawn to the spirit of animals. But she always had a dream of owning her own animal rescue farm.

She sat down for a serious conversation with her partner. They didn't need this five-bedroom home any longer, so why not sell and move to the country, allowing her to fulfill this dream? She felt this sense of newness and purpose course through her veins.

Over the next three years, Tracey would build her dream. With the help of friends and family, her animal rescue became a reality. She now saves hundreds of animals each year, getting them back to health and placing them in their forever homes. This is her legacy. This is something her family can look back on and see their mother's love and compassion.

Full-Circle Framework Component #7: Legacy Building

So, we're here, in this glorious—okay, sometimes sweaty—stage of life where we're supposed to be "reflecting on our life and accomplishments," according to this dude, Erik Erikson. He's the brainy fella who mapped out life like it's a giant board game of *Who Am I?* And here we are, playing the level just before the grand finale: integrity vs. despair. Sounds like the least fun game show ever, right? But stick with me; it's actually pretty juicy.

In the world according to Erik, the last level of life's game is about looking back and thinking, *Did I slay this this thing called life or what?* A high score means you've got a golden ticket to Integrity Land— population: proud, content, and flaunting the silver streaks. Flunk it, and it's a one-way trip to Despairville, where the main activity is kicking yourself for what you could've, would've, or should've done (Cherry, 2022). Boo!

What you need to know is that the big ol' integrity thing isn't just about you. It's about what you're leaving behind, and I'm not talking about your vintage handbag collection. It's about your mark on the world, your essence, and the you-ness that's going to stick around, like that stubborn glitter from the craft project you did back in 2009.

Now, let's talk turkey about this whole legacy business. I mean, we're not ancient pharaohs trying to build pyramids, but we do have this nifty opportunity to craft something that lasts. And no, it's not all about the Benjamins or being the next Oprah. It's about the laughs you shared, the shoulders you offered for others to cry on, and those moments you stood up for what's right—even when your voice shook.

You see, menopause isn't just a time for hot flashes and putting fans in all the places; it's the perfect time to ponder the legacy you want to leave. With our estrogen on vacation, something amazing happens—our self-awareness goes through the roof! Suddenly, we're reevaluating everything. Does my job spark joy? Should I really spend another weekend watching pet videos? Okay, maybe that's still a yes.

It's like a significant shift in priorities has snuck up on us. Suddenly, instead of fretting over raising the next Mozart or climbing the corporate ladder, we're thinking, "How can I sprinkle a little more me in the world?" That could mean mentoring, volunteering, or just spreading good vibes.

And sure, this whole menopause shebang reminds us that we're not immortal—rude awakening, I know. But instead of going all doom and gloom, this is our opportunity to kick it up a notch. We get to decide what memories and wisdom we're going to pass on. It's like, "Hey, world, you're going to remember the sass and class I brought to the table."

What does this mean for you? It means menopause is your runway to take off into a future with purpose and direction. Whether you want to paint, protest, write the next great American novel, or simply be the neighborhood's coolest cookie-baking, advice-giving auntie, this is your time.

Now, go. Shine on, you crazy diamond. Your legacy awaits!

Creating Your Legacy

Oh, honey, sit down and grab your ice pack because, let's face it, we're always five seconds away from a personal summer, and let's

Chapter 8

dish about legacies. I'm not talking about the "written in a dusty old book" kind of legacy. I'm talking about the "I lived, loved, and maybe flashed the mailman during a hot flash" type. Yep, that's the stuff that legends—and legacies—are made of.

Now, you might be thinking, *Legacy? I'm just trying to remember why I walked into the kitchen.* But stick with me. We've lived a few chapters, and it's time we start scribbling in the margins, leaving little notes for those coming after us. How do we do it? Listen up, beautiful, because we're about to rewrite the rulebook on menopausal mischief and meaning.

First, live your legacy. Don't just leave it; live it! Live like you mean it, because if we've learned anything, it's that life doesn't hand out encores. We're gonna sashay into every room like we own the place —because we do. Our presence is our legacy, and we're gonna make it felt. So, throw on that outrageous hat you love, and let's dance in the rain. Why? Because we're sensational, that's why.

Love like your life depends on it. Because, let's face it, those hormonal tides have turned us into the most passionate creatures on this side of a romance novel. Remember when we'd scoff at those sappy movies where they declare undying love in the rain? Well, now we're the ones getting teary-eyed at a well-placed Hallmark card. And why not? Love fiercely, laugh loudly, and squeeze every ounce of joy out of this life.

Keep a journal, because someday someone is going to want to know how you made it through the Great Hormonal Upheaval without committing a crime. It'll be your "Menopausal Musings," detailing every bizarre craving, mood swing, and the time you cried over a puppy video. It's raw, it's real, and it's us.

Become someone's mentor. Remember that younger version of you who thought her 30s were going to be "the end?" Give that girl a giggle and show her that life's just getting started. Pass the torch of your hard-earned wisdom—like never trust a fart during a sneeze after 40.

Pass on your knowledge and share the family stories with your children or anyone willing to listen. Those tales of our mishaps and recoveries are the threads that will stitch the past to the future. They need to know about Aunt Edna's UFO sighting or how you started your business with nothing but a brilliant idea and maybe a restless night epiphany.

Be honest—brutally, beautifully honest. By now, we can spot BS a mile away without our reading glasses on. Our legacy is built on our truth—the good, the bad, and the slightly embarrassing.

Volunteer, because giving back is the new social currency. It's also hotter than any flash we've had, and trust me, we've had our share. It's about sharing our superpowers—whether it's knitting, number-crunching, or making a killer lasagna.

Share your lessons. We've fallen, flailed, and failed, but we always flip our hair and get back up. Let's tell those tales, not just as warnings but as beacons of hope. If we can survive puberty, parenting, and perimenopause, we can survive anything.

Ground your purpose in a greater purpose. Whether it's saving the planet one recycled wine bottle at a time or leading the charge on senior dance-offs, let's make it count.

Give your family the gift of time. Sure, diamonds are nice, but memories? Priceless! Be the legend at family gatherings who starts food fights and has a secret handshake with the grandkids.

Inspire the next generation by being unabashedly you. If that means starting a rock band in your 60s or wearing leopard print as a neutral, so be it.

And lastly, give back. Whether it's wisdom, resources, or time, sprinkle that stuff everywhere like confetti.

Chapter 8

Strong Women Who Have Left a Lasting Legacy

Now, we all know this chapter in our lives can feel like our bodies have turned into some kind of twisted amusement park—complete with the world's most unpredictable rollercoaster—hello, mood swings, the haunted house of hormones, and, of course, the bumper cars of sex drive. But amidst this wacky carnival, guess what? We're still on fire—and I don't just mean the hot flashes.

Let's talk about a few women who didn't just walk through the flames but came out on the other side like fabulous, fierce fire-breathers. First up, our gal Jane Goodall. This woman waltzed into the jungle, sat down with chimps, and changed the game of prima-tology. She is a primatologist and anthropologist whose research on wild chimpanzees revolutionized our understanding of primates and human evolution (Natural History Museum, n.d.). Menopause? Pfft. More like meno-power. She didn't let a little thing like age stop her from hanging out with our primate cousins and showing the world that animals are a lot more like us than we thought.

And then there's Ruth Bader Ginsburg, who was out there busting her butt for gender equality with the tenacity of a superhero—and, let's be honest, with way better collars. Elected to the Supreme Court, she was throwing down major legal precedents while most people her age were throwing in the towel (*Ruth Bader Ginsberg*, 2020). I like to imagine her coolly adjusting her jabot before serving up justice, like it's a tennis match and she's aiming for that sweet, sweet victory.

And can we have a moment of sizzling applause for Maya Angelou? The woman was a poet, dancer, singer, activist, and about five other kinds of amazing. She showed us that words have the power to change the world, and she did it all with a grace that makes me want to stand up a little straighter (Gilliam, 2017).

What's the takeaway from these legendary ladies? They didn't let a little hormone fluctuation or society stop them from leaving legacies that last longer than any "best by" date society tries to slap on us. They wrote, they fought, they researched, and they lived with the kind of passion that we all have boiling inside of us—sometimes quite literally.

And if you think menopause means the end of sexy, then, honey, you haven't been paying attention. We're redefining sexy on our terms. It's about confidence, wit, and that certain *je ne sais quoi* that comes with not having time for anyone's foolishness. We're not invisible; we're invincible.

So, next time you're mourning the loss of your estrogen like it was a beloved pet, remember these women. They didn't slow down; they shifted gears. And they didn't just get through menopause; they harnessed that hormonal rollercoaster and rode it all the way to the Hall of Fame.

Chapter 8 Challenge: Your Legacy Statement

I want you to consider this your playful prompt to pen something a bit more spirited than a grocery list: your legacy statement.

Now, hold on to your espressos, sisters, because we're not talking about carving our names on some old, dusty plaque. No way. We're about to script the spicy, soulful, and sassy saga that is us.

What's a legacy statement, you ask? It's a declaration, your personal press release to the universe, announcing the mark you're going to leave on this wild party called life. And believe me, it's not about being perfect; it's about being present, passionate, and perhaps a pinch peculiar—because, let's face it, normal is just a setting on a dryer.

Chapter 8

Here's how we'll craft this masterpiece, step by step, like a fine cocktail that's both strong and sweet.

Step One: Reflect on Your Values and Passions

Grab a glass of wine or maybe even the whole bottle—we don't judge here—and let's get down to business. What gets your heart racing faster than seeing your favorite actor in a surprise movie cameo? Is it family? Friendship? The feeling when you find an extra fry at the bottom of the bag? Jot these down. These nuggets of gold are the bedrock of your legacy.

Step Two: Consider Your Impact

Imagine the splash you want to make in the pond. Whether it's nurturing a garden, building a business, or being the one who always has the best stories at a party, think about how you want to touch the lives around you. You are the pebble, and the ripples are your legacy. What will they be?

Step Three: Define Your Legacy

In a sentence or two, because brevity is the soul of wit, define your legacy. It might be something like, "She left a sparkle wherever she went, and not just from her glitter nail polish."

Step Four: Articulate Your Legacy Statement

Expand on your zesty little sentence like you're telling the most gripping story at brunch. Make it rich with the values you adore, the change you want to spearhead, and the quirks that make you unmistakably you.

Step Five: Revise and Refine

Think of your legacy statement as a beautiful draft in the hands of a writer who's lived a life rich with plot twists and character development. We might wake up one day and find that what we valued at 35 is now as outdated as shoulder pads and perms. Our statement must be able to shimmy and shake just as we do when our favorite tune comes on.

Revisit your statement like an old friend. Sit down with it over a cup of tea or a glass of wine, and ask, "Darling, how have you grown?" Nurture it as you do your garden or your endless collection of scarves. Trim the excess, add in new blooms, and maybe sprinkle a little glitter on it for good measure.

Step Six: Live Your Legacy

Let's get this legacy party started, shall we? Flip to your favorite notebook—you know, the one with the inspirational quote on the cover—and let the pen do the two-step across the page. After all, if menopause has taught us anything, it's that we're capable of rewriting the script and making it a blockbuster hit.

Write your legacy and live your legacy.

As we look to the future and to the generations of women who will follow in our occasionally unstable footsteps, we leave behind not only our stories but also the power of laughter. It's the kind of legacy that doesn't require a trust fund, just an open heart and the willingness to see the comedy in the chaos.

May our laughter be a beacon for our daughters and their daughters, a torch carried through the dark times and the light, reminding them that strength comes from the ability to not only endure but to find joy in the enduring.

Let's conclude this chapter not with a whimper but with a triumphant roar. We've earned every laugh line etched upon our faces and wear them as badges of honor.

Conclusion

Oh, my radiant, fierce, and fabulous friends, we've shared quite the journey between these pages, haven't we? From sweat-soaked sheets to mood swings that could give a pendulum a run for its money, we've laughed, we've cried, and we've given those pesky menopause myths a kick in the ovaries.

Now, as we reach the end of this crazy ride, which, by the way, is only the beginning of another, let's not forget what we've discovered. Menopause isn't the end of your story. It's a plot twist in your ongoing, fabulous narrative. It's the time when the caterpillar says, "Screw this," breaks out of the cocoon, and starts a tango class. Yep, we're about to dance like everyone's watching, and we don't give a hoot because we've got moves they haven't even seen yet.

The key takeaway? You are the same knockout who turned heads at 20, the powerhouse who built a life at 30, and the heart that held a family together at 40. What's changed? The number? Pfft. Numbers are for bank accounts, not for defining our vibrancy or our worth.

Conclusion

Menopause is not a pause but a play button to the next funky tune. You're not fading into the background; you're the headliner in your show. Sure, our bodies are remixing themselves, but honey, we've always been the masters of reinvention.

Let's raise our glasses and celebrate this journey and the wisdom we've collected like the finest of pearls—wisdom that has come from living, loving, losing, and leaping into the unknown with a parachute woven from our strength.

As you step out into the world, my magnificent midlife queens, do it with a sense of curiosity, excitement, and gratitude. With every hot flash, remember that you're not overheating; you're just on fire, in the best possible way. With every new wrinkle, see a line of a new chapter, one that you are writing with the pen of experience and the ink of resilience.

You are strong, my friend. You are resilient. And you are so capable of navigating this season with grace and poise that you'll make autumn leaves jealous. Now, go ahead. Step into this new chapter with confidence.

It's going to be beautiful, just like you.

But before you go, do a gal a solid, will ya? If you had a laugh, found a compatriot in these pages, or simply enjoyed the ride, drop a review. Share your story, your triumphs, and yes, even those "oops, I peed a little" moments. Your words might just be the light-house for another soul setting sail on the menopause seas.

Thank you!

Now, off you go. Reclaim that sexy, grab your confidence by the reigns, and ride off into that hot flash of a sunset. And remember, you've got so much to offer.

It's time to live out loud. The world isn't ready for you, but that's just too bad. Here you come!

References

Admin. (2017, May 15). *50 Best Sharing Knowledge Quotes - Words of Great Wisdom.* Quotespeak.

Blanchflower, D. G., Graham, C., & Piper, A. (2023). *Happiness and age—resolving the debate.* National Institute Economic Review, 1–18.

Busch, A. (2023, April 6). *Akiko Busch: 'Mrs. Dalloway' shows aging has benefits.* The Atlantic.

Calra, R. (2022, September 18). *Menopause, not an end to youth but beginning of a new phase!!* The Statesman.

Cherry, K. (2022, August 3). *Erik Erikson's stages of psychosocial development.* Very Well Mind.

Cooper, J. (2022, October 26). Breathe A poem by Becky Helmsley - Talking to the Wild | My CMS. *My CMS.*

Davis, A. (2023, June 22). *53 sexual affirmations to build a sex-positive mindset.* Ambitiously Alexa.

18 signs of the menopause you might have missed. (n.d.). HCA Healthcare UK.

English, C. B. B. I. (2022, June 6). *50+ famous quotes about leaving a lasting legacy.* Cake Blog.

Fields, L. (2021, January 7). *8 Interesting facts about Laura Ingalls Wilder.* American Masters.

Gilliam, S. (2017, February 10). *Why Maya Angelou's legacy will never be forgotten.* HelloBeautiful.

Green, A. (2016, December 1). *The incredible story of the woman in the senior freshman meme.* Refinery29.

Haak, E. (2014, June 19). *How a little self-compassion can ease hot flashes.* Prevention.

Hampson, L. (2022, October 18). *New research shows link between menopause and divorce.* The Independent.

Hemsley, R. (n.d.). Poetry by Becky Hemsley. Instagram.

How does menopause affect sexual function? (2022, April 14). Moreland OB-GYN.

Menopause hormones – What are they and how do they change? (2020, October 28). Forth.

Natural History Museum. (n.d.). *A closer look at becoming Jane: Her scientific legacy.* Natural History Museum.

Navigating the menopause: A spiritual perspective. (2023, September 8). Spiritual Quest.

Nuss, H. (2018, April 4). *Aging gracefully and what it means to Helena.* Manor Medical Aesthetics.

Rabin, J. (n.d.). *Women have been shamed and stigmatized over menopause for years.* Northwell Health.

References

Resnick, M. (2014, December 8). *20 amazing life lessons nature has taught us*. Lifehack.

Ruth Bader Ginsberg. (2020, September). CT.gov.

Seaman, A. (2022, April 4). *What we can learn from Julia Child about career second acts*. LinkedIn.

Size of the anti-aging market worldwide 2018-2023. (2018). Statista.

Sharratt, M. (2019, November 9). *The fierce initiation of menopause by Mary Sharratt*. Feminism and Religion.

Tamae Watanabe, 73, smashes own record as oldest woman to climb Mount Everest. (2012, May 19). NBC News.

10 ways to leave a legacy. (2012, October 18). All Pro Dad.

10 ways to reinvent yourself after 50. (2020, July 16). After Fifty Living.

Top 10 symptoms of low estrogen. (2019, February 20). OB/GYN Associates of Alabama.

25 journal prompts for self-discovery for midlife women in menopause. (2023, July 20). Wellness Reset Life Coach.

27 powerful Reinvent Yourself quotes – Better believe it! (n.d.).

Vogel, K. (2021, July 26). *Whether you're 25 or 65, here are 50 quotes about menopause that will resonate with every woman*. Parade.

Warrick, P. (1994, August 9). *Feminists face off in war over menopause*. Los Angeles Times.

Weiss, C. (2019, May 16). *Women's wellness: Menopause misconceptions*. Mayo Clinic.

Weyhrich, D. (n.d.). *How lifestyle changes can impact your menopausal symptoms*. Darin L. Weyhrich, M.D.

Wiseman, E. (2019, May 19). *It's time to talk about the menopause… and freedom at last*. The Guardian.

www.ingramcontent.com/pod-product-compliance
Lightning Source LLC
Chambersburg PA
CBHW060253150626
46553CB00019BA/2109